The Dictionary of
IMMUNOLOGY

The Dictionary of

IMMUNOLOGY

Fourth Edition

W. John Herbert PhD, MRCVS, DVTM

Formerly, Senior Lecturer, Department of Immunology,
University of Glasgow

Peter C. Wilkinson MD, FRSE

Professor, Department of Immunology,
University of Glasgow

David I. Stott BSc, PhD

Senior Lecturer, Department of Immunology,
University of Glasgow

ACADEMIC PRESS

Harcourt Brace & Company, Publishers
London   San Diego   New York
Boston   Sydney   Tokyo   Toronto

Cover illustration

Digitized-colour transmission electron micrograph (TEM) of a human T lymphocyte cell. Here, the
cell has released some of its cytoplasm (at bottom, yellow). The nucleus is coloured purple.

Photograph by R. Roseman. Courtesy of the Science Photo Library.

Typeset by Photo·graphics, Honiton, Devon
Printed and bound in Great Britain by Hartnolls Limited, Bodmin, Cornwall

Preface

In the ten years since the third edition of the *Dictionary of Immunology* was published, dramatic developments have occurred in the science of immunology. Many problems unsolved ten years ago now have answers, especially the central questions about how the specificity of the immune response is determined at the molecular level. During those ten years, molecular biology has made a major impact on immunology both at the conceptual level and at the laboratory bench. The new edition of the Dictionary has been radically revised to bring it in line with what can be described without exaggeration as a culture shift. People are doing different things now and thinking differently from the way they were thinking in 1985.

With insight has come expansion and specialization and we no longer feel that a compact dictionary of the subject can, as earlier editions did, encompass everything from the immunology of invertebrates and domestic animals to the intricacies of the structure of histocompatibility antigens. This edition has, therefore, been trimmed to address the fundamentals from which all applications spring. This has meant omitting many laboratory techniques which have been superseded by more sensitive assays, and omitting details of reagents with specific applications, such as vaccines, unless they help to illuminate some basic immunological concept. Regrettably we have also had to omit some definitions of historical importance.

The restructuring of the Dictionary has led to the replacement of over a third of the previous entries and the revision of those remaining. We have included a large number of new entries, especially to cover cell membrane proteins, cytokines and other molecules of major interest. We have not included many entries on cell signalling, since this is a subject in which it is still not clear which mechanisms are central to control of immune function. Overall we have kept the book to about its original size: it was always intended to be a volume that could be consulted readily in the hand.

Without the willing assistance of colleagues in the University of Glasgow and elsewhere, this revision would never have been possible. Colleagues from many places have helped or advised with definitions and their willingness to do so has, we hope, been a measure of the esteem in which previous editions have been held. The names of contributors who wrote new definitions are listed overleaf. Many colleagues wrote definitions for earlier editions and were acknowledged there. Their work forms the foundation on which this edition is based. We also especially thank Dr Neil Barclay (University of Oxford) who allowed us to use, and provided copies of, illustrations from *The Leucocyte Antigen Factsbook* (Academic Press). The figures were prepared in the Department of Medical Illustration at the Western Infirmary, Glasgow. We hope that this edition will prove as useful as earlier ones were.

John Herbert
Peter Wilkinson
David Stott

Major contributors

Dr Elizabeth R. Holme
Dr Charles McSharry
Dr Allan M. Mowat

All of the Department of Immunology,
University of Glasgow

Other contributors

Professor J. A. Bradley

Fraser Darling

Nancy Henderson

Professor F. Y. Liew

Dr I. Newman

Dr A. J. Wilkinson

Departments of Surgery and
Immunology, University of Glasgow
Department of Clinical Veterinary
Medicine, University of Cambridge
Department of Immunology,
University of Glasgow (Royal
Infirmary)
Department of Immunology,
University of Glasgow
Department of Immunology,
University of Glasgow
Department of Chemistry, University
of York

Figures

Tables

Arrangement of the Entries

The entries are listed in alphabetical order of the separate words, thus bringing all those with the same first word together. Hyphens have been treated as spaces in the alphabetization.

Greek letters, where they form the initial character, have been placed as if they were spelled out in English, i.e. 'α' is placed as 'alpha'. They are spelled out on their first appearance and the Greek alphabet is printed in Appendix Table 3.

Synonyms, if any, are shown in parentheses after headwords. Some of these are older usages.

Cross References

We have cross-referenced extensively (shown as **_bold italic_**) with the intention that readers will never wonder whether or not it is worth searching the dictionary for a word or phrase. Cross references are shown only once in any entry.

The cross references are usually to the exact headword (ignoring plurals) but where this would lead to clumsy construction or additional explanation, we have cross referenced a related part of speech to that of the actual headword so as to lead the reader to the relevant area, e.g. _phagocytic_ would, we hope, lead to **phagocyte** and **phagocytosis**.

In a very few cases the cross reference has a superscript numeral attached. This indicates that the entry has several definitions which are very different from each other; the numeral directs the reader to the part intended e.g. _challenge_[2].

Headword Under Which Defined

Where there is a choice, usually between the spelt-out and abbreviated form, we have tried to place the definition under the term that is in more general, usually colloquial, use.

T and B Cells/T and B Lymphocytes

These terms are used interchangeably in speech and text – we have followed this informal usage rather than use the pedantically correct _T lymphocyte_ or _B lymphocyte_ throughout.

Abbreviations Used in the Entries

Many abbreviations and acronyms for substances and activities of immunological interest will be found as headwords or synonyms in the text. A list of 'Standard abbreviations' for immunological materials is printed as Appendix Table 1. Other abbreviations used in the text are:

cf.   compare
e.g.   for example
esp.   especially
Gell and Coombs   *Clinical Aspects of Immunology* (1963). 1st Edn. Oxford, Blackwell Scientific Publications.
H & E stain   haematoxylin and eosin stain
i.e.   that is to say
inter alia   amongst other things
mm   millimetre
nm   nanometre (millimicron, mμ)
q.v.   which see (where used indicates important extension to the definition)
®   Word known or thought to be a proprietary name. The inclusion of any other proprietary name without such indication is not to be taken as a representation by the editors or publisher that it is not subject to proprietary rights
Syn.   synonym
μm   micrometre (μ or micron)
viz.   namely

A

a Prefixed abbreviation for 'anti' used to mean *'antibody* against' as in 'aCD3' (antibody to *CD3*).

ab Abbreviation for *antibody*.

aberrant clone See *forbidden clone* (preferred term).

ABO blood group substances Soluble substances bearing *ABO blood group system* specificity. Present in human mucous secretions, e.g. ovarian cyst fluid, gastric juice, saliva, etc. of 80% of humans (termed 'secretors'). They are high molecular weight glycopeptides with a high-peptide-content backbone and oligosaccharide side chains bearing ABO *epitopes* identical to those of the erythrocytes of the same individual.

ABO blood group system One of the human *blood group* systems. It is the most important in blood transfusion serology because *natural antibodies* against ABO blood group *antigens* occur in the *plasma*. Humans belong to one of four groups: A, B, AB and O; the red cells of each group carry respectively the A antigen, the B antigen, both A and B antigens, or neither antigen. The *antibodies* in their plasma are specific for those ABO antigens not present on the red cells of the bearer, e.g. persons of group A have antibodies to the B antigen, as shown in Table A1.

Table A1. Human ABO blood group system

Blood group (phenotype)	Antigen on cells	Antibody in plasma
A	A	anti B
B	B	anti A
AB	A and B	neither
O	neither	anti A and anti B

absorption In immunology the term refers to the use of reagents to remove *antigens* or *antibodies* from a mixture. Used to remove unwanted possibly *cross reacting antibodies* from an *antiserum* to make it more specific. Accomplished by adding antigen and then removing the antigen–antibody complex formed. Cf. *adsorption*.

accessory cell Cell that is essential for initiating *T cell* dependent *immune responses* usually by presenting *antigen*, bound to *class II MHC antigen* molecules, to *CD4*+ T lymphocytes (see also *antigen-presenting cell*). Accessory cells include class II MHC+ *mononuclear phagocytes, dendritic cells* and *B lymphocytes* but, under certain conditions other cell types can express class II MHC antigen molecules and may act as accessory cells.

acquired immune deficiency syndrome See *AIDS*.

acquired immunity *Immunity[1]* that develops as a specific response to an *antigenic* substance or organism. Cf. *native immunity* and *non-specific immunity*.

activated lymphocyte Any *lymphocyte* in an active state of proliferation or differentiation.

activated macrophage *Macrophage* with increased functional activity induced by a stimulating agent. The term was first used of macrophages that, following *in vivo* injection of infectious agents such as *Listeria monocytogenes*, differentiated to become more efficient killers of the injected bacteria than macrophages from untreated animals. Activation in this system is *T lymphocyte*-dependent and is mediated by release of macrophage activating factors such as gamma interferon (*IFN-γ*). The term activation is often also used to refer to the enhancement of other macrophage functions. It should probably only be used with a qualification defining the experimental system under study.

active immunity Protection due to development of an *immune response* in an individual following stimulation with *antigen*, e.g. in a *vaccine* or during infection. Cf. *passive immunity*.

active immunization Stimulation of an individual's *immune responses* in order to confer protection against disease. Effected by exposure to *protective antigens* either during the course of infection (which may be subclinical) or by *vaccination*. The protection effected takes a week or more to develop, but is then long lasting and rapidly revived by a *booster dose* (see *immunological memory*). Cf. *passive immunization*.

acute lymphoblastic leukaemia (ALL) Leukaemia of *lymphocyte* precursors, usually of *B cells*. The commonest form of leukaemia in children. The most frequent form is pre-B ALL (see *pre-B lymphocyte*). These cells have B cell markers *CD19* and *CD22*, are *TdT+*, often *CD10+*, and have rearranged *immunoglobulin genes*. Cytoplasmic μ chains (see *heavy chain*) may be present. More rarely *membrane immunoglobulin* (mIg) is present: if so the term B-ALL is used. Acute *T cell* leukaemia (T-ALL) is uncommon. These cells are TdT+, CD7+, have rearranged *TCR* genes and cytoplasmic *CD3*, but do not express surface T cell markers, thus resemble *double-negative thymocytes*.

acute myeloblastic leukaemia (acute myeloid leukaemia) Leukaemia in which the predominant cell type is myeloblast-like. The leukaemia probably arises from *myeloid cell series* precursors or from pluripotent *stem cells*. *Immunoglobulin genes* and *TCR* genes are not rearranged and *B cell* and *T cell* markers are absent. Surface CD13 and CD33 are usually present and are used as markers.

acute phase reactants Non-*antibody* proteins synthesized by hepatocytes (liver cells) and, to a lesser extent, by *macrophages*, which appear in increased quantities in *plasma* in response to *cytokines* (e.g. *IL-6* and *IL-1*) induced by tissue damage or infection. They include *C reactive protein*, fibrinogen, certain *complement* components, α1-antitrypsin and α1-acid glycoprotein (orosomucoid). Functions still debatable.

acute phase serum Serum collected in the acute phase of an infectious disease. Cf. *convalescent serum*.

acute respiratory distress syndrome (ARDS) Bilateral patchy consolidation of the lungs occurring as a complication of severe injury. Caused by increased alveolar leakiness resulting in pulmonary oedema with fluid rich in protein. The mortality is high. The mechanism is unknown but may be caused by release of mediators such as *IL-8* by *alveolar macrophages* initiating an inflammatory infiltrate.

ADA deficiency See *adenosine deaminase deficiency*.

ADCC See *antibody-dependent cell-mediated cytotoxicity*.

Addison's disease Adrenal cortical hypofunction, the commonest form of which is due to autoimmune damage (see *autoimmunity*). *Autoantibodies* to adrenal cortical *antigens* (steroid hormone producing cells) are present in the *serum*. These include autoantibodies to corticotrophin receptors, which block ACTH-mediated adrenal stimulation. Experimental allergic adrenalitis has been produced by injecting adrenal tissue into experimental animals.

addressin An imprecise term used to refer to the structures on a vascular endothelial cell that are recognized by *homing receptors* on *leucocytes* (particularly *lymphocytes*) thus allowing specific entry of leucocytes into a tissue in, for example, *lymphocyte recirculation* or inflammation. The 'address' of a tissue is probably in reality quite complex, involving several selective *adhesion molecules* rather than any single one.

adenosine deaminase (ADA) deficiency An enzyme defect inherited as an autosomal recessive trait. Presents as a form of *SCID* in infants with deficiencies of both *B lymphocyte* precursors and *T lymphocyte* precursors. Adenosine deaminase is abundant in normal *lymphocytes* and in the *thymus* and its lack causes failure of adenosine metabolism and accumulation of toxic metabolites in lymphocyte precursors.

adhesion molecules See Table A2.

adjuvant Substance injected with *antigens* (usually mixed with them but sometimes given prior to or following the antigen) which non-specifically enhances or modifies the *immune response* to that antigen. Thus *antibody* production or the reactions of *cell-mediated immunity* are more vigorous than would be the case were the antigen injected without adjuvant. In addition, the response may be modified qualitatively, e.g. antibodies of different *immunoglobulin classes* may be stimulated. See *aluminium adjuvants*, *complete Freund's adjuvant*, *incomplete Freund's adjuvant*, *ISCOM*, *lipopolysaccharide* and *mycobacterial adjuvants*.

adjuvant arthritis Clinical abnormality following injection of *complete Freund's adjuvant*, without an added *antigen*, into experimental animals especially rats. Also inducible with *heat shock protein*-65 from *Mycobacterium tuberculosis*. Characterized by inflammatory lesions in joints and periarticular tissues particularly those of the extremities and tail.

adjuvant disease See *adjuvant arthritis*.

adjuvant granuloma *Granuloma* that forms at the site of injection of adjuvants, e.g. *complete Freund's adjuvant* and *aluminium adjuvants*.

adjuvanticity The ability of a substance to enhance or modify an *immune response* in a non-specific manner (see *adjuvant*).

adoptive immunity *Passive immunity* transmitted, not by *antibody* but by *lymphocytes*. See *cell-mediated immunity*.

adoptive transfer *Passive transfer* of immunity by transferring *lymphocytes* from a *primed* donor to a non-immune recipient (see *non-immune animal*).

adsorption Non-specific, non-covalent, binding of soluble substances (in immunology usually *antibodies* or *antigens*), to the surfaces of cells or inert particles. E.g. If red cells to which an antigen has become adsorbed are exposed to the relevant antibody they will show *agglutination*. Cf. *absorption*.

adult T cell leukaemia/lymphoma A form of leukaemia especially common in Japan and the Caribbean caused by infection with the virus HTLV-1 (human *T cell* leukaemia virus-1).

AET-rosette test A test for human *T lymphocytes* using 2-aminoethylisothiouridium bromide-treated sheep erythrocytes which bind to *CD2* on T lymphocytes to form rosettes. These rosettes are more stable than E rosettes formed using untreated sheep erythrocytes (see *E-rosette forming cell*). Commonly used to purify *B cells* by separating out rosetted T cells.

affinity A thermodynamic expression of the strength of interaction or binding between two entities, e.g. between an *antigen-binding site* and *epitope*, and thus, of the stereochemical compatibility between them. As such it is expressed as the equilibrium or association constant (K litres mole^{-1}) for the *antigen–antibody* interaction but, since there is usually a heterogeneity of affinities within a population of antibody molecules of defined specificity it is, at best, an average value referred to as the 'mean intrinsic association constant'. The term affinity is most accurately applied to interactions involving simple, uniform determinants, e.g. *haptens*, thus obviating the difficulty of considering heterogeneous determinants on the same molecule.

Table A2. Adhesion molecules. This table only includes adhesion molecules known to be of importance in the immune system and for which there is an entry in the Dictionary. Further details will be found under individual entries

Molecule	Distribution	Ligand
Selectins		
L-selectin	Most leucocytes	*GlyCAM-1*, sialyl glycoproteins
E-selectin	*Cytokine*-activated vascular endothelium	Sialyl Lewis x
P-selectin	Storage granules in vascular endothelium and *platelets*	Sialyl Lewis x
CD44	Many leucocytes	Hyaluronate
Integrins		
β_2-integrins		
CD11a/CD18 (LFA-1)	Most leucocytes	*ICAM-1, -2, -3*
CD11b/CD18 (MAC-1) (CR3)	Mono, MΦ, PMN; NK	*ICAM-1*, iC3b
CD11c/CD18 (p150:95) (CR4)	Mono, MΦ, PMN, NK, DC	*ICAM-1*, iC3b
β_1-integrins		
CD49d/CD29 (VLA-4)	T, Mono, Bas, Eos	*VCAM-1*
Other integrins		
$\alpha_4\beta_7$	T	*MAd-CAM-1*
$\alpha_E\beta_7$ ($\alpha_{HML}\beta_7$; see *HML-1*)	T	
Ig superfamily		
ICAM-1 (CD54)	Vascular endothelium. Inducible on many cells	*LFA-1*
ICAM-2 (CD102)	Vascular endothelium. Inducible on many cells	*LFA-1*
ICAM-3 (CD50)	Most leucocytes	*LFA-1*
VCAM-1 (CD106)	Vascular endothelium, MΦ, DC	VLA-4
CD2 (LFA-2)	T	*LFA-3*
LFA-3 (CD58)	Most cells	CD2
MAd-CAM-1	Mucosal *high endothelial venules*	$\alpha_4\beta_7$
CD31 (PECAM)	Many leucocytes, vascular endothelium	
GlyCAM-1	*High endothelial venules*	L-*selectin*

Abbreviations: Bas = *basophil leucocyte*; DC = *dendritic cell*; Eos = *eosinophil leucocyte*; Mono = *monocyte*; MΦ = *macrophage*; NK = *NK cell*; PMN = *neutrophil leucocyte*; T = *T cell*.

affinity labelling Immunochemical method of identifying peptides located in the *antigen-binding site*. *Antibody* is treated with a chemically reactive *hapten* which binds specifically to the antigen-binding site and, more slowly, bonds covalently to amino acid residues in close proximity. The antibody is then hydrolysed and the peptide fragments bound to the hapten separated and identified.

affinity maturation Increase in *affinity* of *antibody* occurring during the immune response, especially between a *primary immune response* and a *secondary immune response*. This is due to selection of high affinity *B cell* clones under conditions of limiting *antigen* concentration. The high affinity clones arise as a result of *somatic hyper-mutation* of V_H *region* and V_L *region* genes during proliferation of B cells in *germinal centres*.

ag Abbreviation for *antigen*.

agammaglobulinaemia Absence of *immunoglobulin*, see *hypogammaglobu-linaemia*.

agglutination Clumping of particulate *antigens*, e.g. red cells, bacteria, etc. by reaction with specific *antibody* which forms bridges between *epitopes* on contiguous particles. As agglutination is easily visible, it forms the basis of many tests, especially those used in clinical diagnosis.

agglutinin (1) An *antibody* that reacts with surface *antigens* of particles, e.g. red cells and bacteria, to agglutinate them. See *agglutination*. (2) Any substance, not necessarily antibody, capable of agglutinating particles, e.g. *lectin*.

agranulocytosis Pathological fall in the level of circulating *neutrophil leucocytes* resulting from depression of myelo-poiesis. It results in a lowered resistance to bacterial infection, and often presents as a severe pharyngitis (agranulocytic angina). Death may follow from septi-caemia, meningitis, etc. or myelopoiesis may be resumed and recovery follow. Can develop without known cause or following administration of certain cyto-toxic drugs and also as an idiosyncratic response to normally harmless doses of various chemicals or drugs, e.g. chlor-amphenicol.

AIDS (acquired immune deficiency syndrome) Human disease caused by progressive destruction of protective *cell-mediated immunity* as a result of infection with the human immunodefic-iency virus (*HIV*). The virus binds to membrane *CD4* and infects cells, chiefly *helper T lymphocytes*, or *mononuclear phagocytes*, which carry that protein. When the count of CD4+ cells reaches very low levels (less than 200 per mm^3 in blood), usually several years after

infection, patients present with any of a wide variety of repeated, severe, and often fatal opportunistic infections of which *Pneumocystis carinii pneumonia* is the most prominent. There is also an increased incidence of a rare skin tumour, Kaposi's sarcoma. AIDS is not a clearly defined entity and manifests itself differently in different patient groups and in different geographical locations though the prognosis is poor in all groups.

AIDS-related complex (ARC) A term describing the clinical signs and symp-toms associated with the terminal stages of *HIV* infection. These may include dementia, Kaposi's sarcoma, *B cell* lym-phoma, *Pneumocystis carinii pneu-monia*, pneumonia due to atypical mycobacteria and other opportunistic infections. This term is replaced by stag-ing of the disease progression of HIV infection according to criteria defined by the CDC (Center for Disease Control, Atlanta, USA) or WHO (in Europe), based on increasing severity of clinical presentation and *CD4+* lymphocyte count.

albumin The major protein component of *plasma* (and *serum*). Overall negative charge at neutral pH therefore migrates rapidly to anode on electrophoresis relative to the *globulins* (e.g. *immunoglobulins*) as in *immunoelec-trophoresis*.

alkaline phosphatase/anti alkaline phosphatase staining See *APAAP*.

allelic exclusion An exception to the rule that genes (or alleles) are expressed by both of the chromosomes of the pair that bear them. The *heavy chain* and *light chain* genes of *immunoglobulins* are examples of this exception in that only one allele is expressed by them. Thus, in animals heterozygous for immunoglobulin *allotypes*, *B lympho-cytes* express only one of the allotypes not both.

allergen Antigenic substance (see *antigen*) capable of provoking an *IgE* antibody response. In common usage the term is restricted to substances, e.g.

house dust mite (*Dermatophagoides pteronyssinus*), pollens and dander (see *dander antigen*), that combine with the IgE *antibody* to provoke *allergic responses* in *atopic* subjects.

allergic alveolitis Inflammation of the gas-exchanging part of the lungs consisting of an infiltrate mainly of *lymphocytes*. Caused by inhaling aerosols of organic particulates of about 1 μm diameter which are small enough to penetrate and sediment in the terminal airways. The main syndromes include *bird fancier's lung* (frequently pigeons or budgerigars), and *farmer's lung*. The disease process is thought to involve *antibody* activity against the soluble components of the aerosols and a granulomatous (see *granuloma*) response to the particulates.

allergic encephalomyelitis See *experimental allergic encephalomyelitis*.

allergic response An *immune response* characterized by tissue damage due to *immediate hypersensitivity* following exposure to *allergens*.

allergic rhinitis Exudative inflammation of the nasal passage occurring in *atopic* persons in contact with airborne *allergen* to which they are sensitive. Caused by local release of vasoactive substances in an *immediate hypersensitivity* reaction. Seasonal allergic rhinitis is a feature of the pollen sensitivity 'hay fever', whereas perennial rhinitis is a feature of sensitivity to the house dust mite *Dermatophagoides pteronyssinus*.

allergy A synonym for *hypersensitivity* especially of *immediate hypersensitivity* type (*type I hypersensitivity reaction*), thus with implication of immunologically induced tissue damage. The term was originally introduced by von Pirquet in 1906 to mean altered host reactivity to an *antigen* but it no longer holds this meaning.

alloantigens Different (allelic) forms of an *antigen* coded for at the same gene locus in all individuals of a species. E.g. some *histocompatibility antigens* are coded for at the same locus but vary between individuals.

alloantiserum An *antiserum* directed against *antigens* of another animal of the same species and raised in that species. E.g. a serum made in one *inbred strain* of a species against another inbred strain of the same species.

allogeneic (allogenic) Genetically dissimilar within the same species. See also *transplantation terminology*.

allograft Graft exchanged between two genetically dissimilar individuals of the same species, e.g. members of an outbred population, or of two different inbred strains. Cf. *syngeneic*.

allograft rejection *Immunological rejection* of an *allograft* due to a specific *immune response* mounted by the recipient's tissues against the graft. Caused by *incompatibility* of *histocompatibility antigens* between donor and recipient. The rejection is essentially due to *cell-mediated immunity* and is characterized by infiltration of the graft by *lymphocytes*. *Antibody* is usually of less importance.

allotope (allotypic determinant) The structural region of a protein that distinguishes it from the same protein in another individual of the same species.

allotype Serologically identifiable difference between protein molecules that is inherited as an allele of a single genetic locus. Many allotypes have been correlated with amino acid substitutions in the *heavy chains* and *light chains* of *immunoglobulins*, e.g. the *Gm allotypes* and Km allotypes. The *epitope* formed by these amino acids is known as the *allotope*. Allotopes can be found in both the *constant regions* and *variable regions* of immunoglobulins.

allotypic determinant See *allotope*.

α (alpha) See *a*. This is sometimes used instead of 'a' as a prefixed abbreviation for 'anti'.

α chain disease Rare *paraproteinaemia* described in subjects of eastern Mediterranean origin in which there is an infiltrative *lymphoma* especially of the intestine, associated with malabsorption. Abnormal *plasma cells* are present which manufacture only α chains (i.e. *heavy chain* of *IgA*) but no *light chains*. The N-terminal sequences of these α chains are normal but there is a deletion extending from part of the *variable region* through most of the $C_\alpha 1$ *immunoglobulin domain* so that the cysteine residue involved in cross-linking to light chains is missing (see also *γ chain disease* and *heavy chain disease*).

$\alpha_4\beta_7$ (alpha₄beta₇; LPAM-1; leucocyte-Peyer's patch adhesion molecule-1) An *integrin superfamily* molecule present on a proportion of *T lymphocytes*, which binds to the mucosal addressin *MAd-CAM-1*, thus allowing selective homing of *lymphocytes* to mucosal tissues.

alternative pathway (alternate pathway) A pathway by which complement component *C3* is cleaved and *C5–C9* formed without a requirement for *C1*, *C2* or *C4*. Can be activated by bacterial *endotoxin* in the absence of specific *antibody*, and by polysaccharides from various fungal or bacterial sources, and by human *IgA*. See also *Factor B, Factor D̄, properdin* and see Figure A1.

alternative pathway C3 convertase A complex of *C3b*, cleaved *Factor B* (Bb) and *properdin* (C3bBbP) which cleaves *C3* to *C3a* and C3b. C3bBb is an unstable convertase with a short half life which is stabilized by properdin. The C3b produced is essential for the positive feedback loop which forms the *alternative pathway* thus allowing further production of the alternative pathway convertase.

aluminium adjuvants Compounds of aluminium, e.g. aluminium hydroxide gel, aluminium phosphate, aluminium sulphate and alums such as ammonium alum $(NH_4)_2SO_4.Al_2(SO_4)_3$ and potassium alum, that strongly adsorb (see *adsorption*) protein antigens from a solution to form a precipitate. When injected into an animal these precipitates form a depot from which the antigen is slowly released. See also *adjuvant* and *adjuvant granuloma*.

alveolar macrophage A *mononuclear phagocyte* found loosely attached to the walls of pulmonary alveoli and derived from circulating *monocytes* which mature *in situ*. They appear early in lung development and are metabolically adapted to a high pO₂ and to the presence of pulmonary surfactant which they remove by *phagocytosis* giving rise to characteristic cytoplasmic 'myelin

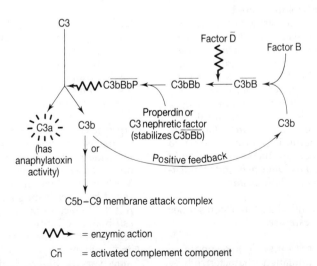

Figure A1. Alternative complement pathway.

figures'. They also remove particles including microorganisms that reach the alveoli. They are normally *immunosuppressive* for *T cells* due to their constitutive release of *prostaglandins* (PGE$_2$) and *platelet activating factor* (PAF). In chronic inflammation they may differentiate into *epithelioid cells* and giant cells producing proteolytic enzymes, chemotactic factors (*IL-8*) and growth factors for fibroblasts (PDGF). They are strongly *class II MHC antigen* and *LFA-1* positive.

aly A mutation in an *inbred strain* of mouse with *immunodeficiency*. These mice fail to develop *lymph nodes* and *Peyer's patches* but other *lymphoid tissues* appear normal.

Am marker An *allotype* of human *IgA2* existing in two forms: A2m(1) and A2m(2). In IgA2m(1) the *light chains* are linked together by a C-terminal disulphide bridge and are not covalently bound to the *heavy chains* owing to the absence of the corresponding cysteine residue in the α chain. In IgA2m(2) the cysteine residues are present in the α chain and are able to form the normal H–L disulphide bridge, see Figure I1.

amyloidosis Disease characterized by deposition of insoluble protein fibrils in a variety of tissues, often leading to failure of affected organs. Two forms of systemic amyloidosis predominate: (a) Reactive amyloidosis which is characterized by fibrils derived from the acute phase protein (see *acute phase reactants*) named serum amyloid protein A (SAA). This form is associated with chronic inflammatory diseases e.g. *rheumatoid arthritis*. (b) Immunocytic amyloidosis in which the fibrils are derived from the *light chains* of *immunoglobulin*. This form is associated with extensive production of free light chains, as in *myelomatosis* and *Waldenström's macroglobulinaemia*.

ANAE (α-naphthyl acetate esterase) See *non-specific esterase*.

anamnestic response (1) Response to antigenic stimulation characterized by production of large amounts of *antibody* against apparently unrelated *antigens*. (2) Unexpectedly powerful antibody response (of *secondary immune response* type) following what is assumed to be an initial administration of antigen. See *heteroclitic antibody*.

anaphylactic shock See *anaphylaxis*.

anaphylactoid reaction An acute shock syndrome resembling *anaphylactic shock* but not caused by an *immunological reaction*. Amongst the substances that may produce this on inoculation are anaesthetic agents and X-ray contrast media. These cause the liberation of large amounts of *histamine* and other *vascular permeability factors* perhaps as a consequence of direct effects on *mast cells* or activation of *complement*. See also *pseudoallergic reaction*.

anaphylatoxins A group of substances, mediators of inflammation, produced in serum during activation of the *complement* cascade (see *C3*, *C4* and *C5*). Anaphylatoxins act indirectly to increase vascular permeability by causing *mast cell* degranulation and *histamine* release. Thus when injected into animals they produce symptoms similar to those of *systemic anaphylaxis*. Anaphylatoxin activity is located in the low molecular weight fragments *C3a* and *C5a* (also *C4a*) that are formed and released after cleavage of C3, C5 and C4.

anaphylatoxin inactivator An enzyme (carboxypeptidase-N) that cleaves the C-terminal arginine from *C5a*, *C3a* and C4a and converts them to C5a$_{desArg}$ C3a$_{desArg}$ and C4a$_{desArg}$, thus causing the loss of *anaphylatoxin* activity. Present in normal human *serum*.

anaphylaxis A severe generalized form of *immediate hypersensitivity* due to the widespread effects of *histamine* and other *vascular permeability factors*. Mechanism identical to that of other *type I hypersensitivity reactions*, i.e. the result of reaction of *antigen* with *mast cell*-bound *IgE* antibody and subsequent release of *vascular permeability factors* and inflammatory substances. Symptoms vary in different species. In man peripheral circulatory failure, hypotension, bronchoconstriction and urticaria are seen. Severe cases can be fatal, especially following intravenous injection of antigen, e.g. anaesthetic agents or suxamethonium; after bee or wasp stings; or after ingestion of foodstuffs, especially peanuts (groundnuts), in sensitized subjects. These reactions are rare.

ANCA See *anti neutrophil cytoplasmic antibody*.

anergy (clonal anergy) Failure of *lymphocytes* that have been *primed* by an *antigen* to respond on second contact with the antigen. Occurs in both *T lymphocytes* and *B lymphocytes* but the term is used particularly of the unresponsiveness that follows when T cells bind to antigen that is presented inappropriately, e.g. in the absence of costimulatory signals. Normally, these signals are provided by contact of the T cell with *costimulatory molecules* other than the *class II MHC antigen*–peptide complex on an *antigen-presenting cell*, but certain 'non-professional' accessory class II MHC antigen+ cells may present antigen without costimulation, leading to anergy.

ANF See *anti nuclear antibody*.

ankylosing spondylitis A chronic inflammatory disease affecting chiefly the spine. Strongly associated with HLA-B27 (see *HLA class I locus*).

annexin Synonym for *lipocortin*. The family of related lipocortins is termed the annexin family.

anti-D *Antibody* against the D antigen of the *Rhesus blood group system*. The commonest and most important antibody formed by the maternal tissues in Rhesus incompatibility. Anti-D can be given within 36 hours of parturition to prevent *isoimmunization* of the mother.

anti globulin test See *antiglobulin test*.

anti I *Antibody* against the I antigen, a *blood group* antigen found on most adult human erythrocytes, A *cold antibody* with this specificity is found as an *autoantibody* in certain cases of cold

antibody type haemolytic anaemia and also in *Mycoplasma pneumoniae* infections.

anti idiotype antibody *Antibody* that binds selectively to a particular *idiotope* or set of idiotopes. Usually produced by *immunizing* an animal with a *monoclonal antibody* (i.e. immunoglobulin) obtained from a member of the same species or by *absorption* of an *antiserum* with *immunoglobulin* that does not bear the idiotope of the immunoglobulin used for immunization.

anti idiotype vaccine A *vaccine* in the form of an *antibody* directed against an idiotypic determinant (see *idiotype*) of another antibody. Antibodies are first raised against a pathogen (Ab1); a second antibody (Ab2) is then raised against the idiotope of the first antibody, i.e. an *anti idiotype antibody*. Some of these Ab2 molecules may have *paratopes* (*antigen-binding sites*) similar to the *epitope* on the pathogen recognised originally by the first antibody, the *internal image*. Immunization of individuals with Ab2 provokes the production of a third antibody (Ab3) against Ab2 and the pathogen. Thus, this procedure vaccinates individuals with antibody instead of *antigen*. The vaccines are highly specific but weak immunogenically. See also *network theory*.

anti neutrophil cytoplasmic antibody (ANCA) *Antibody* to granular components of the human *neutrophil leucocyte* cytoplasm. Two patterns of reactivity are clinically important. 'Cytoplasmic' (C)ANCA results from antibodies binding proteinase 3 and is a diagnostic marker for *Wegener's granulomatosis*. 'Perinuclear' (P)ANCA results from antibodies predominantly to myeloperoxidase and lactoferrin in granules that are attracted to the nuclear membrane during the fixation procedure. (P)ANCA is associated with renal vasculitis, rheumatic and collagen vascular disorders.

anti nuclear antibody *Autoantibody* directed against constituents of cell nuclei. Demonstrable by *immunofluo-*

rescence and present in sera of patients with *systemic lupus erythematosus, Sjögren's disease,* mixed connective tissue disease, scleroderma, and also sometimes in *rheumatoid arthritis.* Different anti nuclear antibodies occur that react with specific nuclear components, e.g. DNA, RNA, RNA-protein, histone and non-histone proteins, giving typical fluorescent staining patterns. Occasionally they are tissue specific, e.g. react with only *polymorphonuclear leucocyte* nuclei (see *tissue specific antigen*).

anti venom (antivenene; antivenin) A therapeutic *antiserum* containing antitoxic *antibodies* capable of specifically neutralizing the venom of one or more kinds of snake or poisonous arthropod.

antibody Protein with the molecular properties of an *immunoglobulin* q.v. and capable of specific combination with *antigen*. Carries *antigen-binding sites* that bind non-covalently with the corresponding *epitope*. Antibodies are produced in the body by the cells of the *B lymphocyte* series and are secreted by *plasma cells*, in response to stimulation by antigen.

antibody combining site See *antigen-binding site*.

antibody deficiency syndrome *Immunodeficiency* either genetically determined or secondary to other diseases. Characterized by low serum *immunoglobulin* levels and failure to produce *antibody* normally on *antigenic* challenge. One, two or all three of the major classes of immunoglobulin (*IgG, IgA* and *IgM*) may be deficient. May exist in the presence of normal *cell-mediated immunity.* See *common variable immunodeficiency, IgA deficiency, IgG subclass deficiencies, X-linked agammaglobulinaemia* and *X-linked hyper-IgM syndrome*.

antibody-dependent cell-mediated cytotoxicity (ADCC) Killing of target cells by *lymphocytes* or other *leucocytes* which carry, bound to *Fc receptors, antibody* specific for the target cell. Thus dependent on an *immunological response* to the target cells, though the killer cell may not be the cell that made the antibody, but rather a passive carrier of antibody, e.g. *neutrophil leucocytes* and *NK cells* act in ADCC.

antibody excess Presence in a mixture of an amount of *antibody* sufficient to combine with all of the *epitopes* in that mixture and still to leave free, uncombined antibody molecules. Under such conditions, no uncombined epitopes remain available for cross links between adjacent *antigen* molecules to be made (see *lattice hypothesis*). Therefore *soluble complexes*, rather than precipitates, are formed. Seen especially in *precipitin tests* of the tube or *gel diffusion test* type.

antibody half-life A measure of the average time of survival of any given *antibody* molecule after its synthesis. In practice, the time taken for the elimination of 50% of a measured dose of antibody from the body of the animal. The various *immunoglobulin classes* have different half-lives, thus the half-life of antibody will vary according to immunoglobulin class.

antigen A molecule that elicits a specific *immune response* when introduced into the tissues of an animal. This may take the form of *antibody* production, or *cell-mediated immunity,* or the animal may show specific *immunological tolerance.* If antigens are to stimulate a response, they must normally be foreign to the animal to which they are administered (but see *autoantigen*). Most antigens are proteins, peptides or polysaccharides. Macromolecular antigens bear small *epitopes* that can be recognized on the intact antigen molecule by specific antibody but *T lymphocytes* recognize only peptides derived from processed protein antigens (see *antigen processing*). Note that any single protein or polysaccharide molecule may bear multiple epitopes. Ultimately the definition of an antigen is arbitrary since specific responsiveness is a property of the host tissues, not of the injected substance.

antigen adjuvant (immunological adjuvant) Term sometimes used to distinguish *adjuvants* used in immunology from those used in other fields, e.g. pharmacology.

antigen–antibody complex See *immune complex*.

antigen-binding capacity A primary measure of the total amount of *antibody* that is available to combine with an *antigen*. It is a measure of the total effective antibody, of all *immunoglobulin classes*, that is present.

antigen-binding site The region of an *antibody* molecule or T cell receptor (*TCR*) that combines specifically with the corresponding *epitope*. In antibody molecules it is present on the *Fab fragment*. The *heavy chains* and *light chains* both participate and the binding site is formed from loops formed by the *variable regions* of both chains. These loops contain the *hypervariable regions* which make intimate contact with the epitope. *Framework region* amino acid side chains are also sometimes involved. Similarly, the antigen binding site of the T cell receptor is formed by the variable region domains of the paired αβ or γδ chains. T cell epitopes are presented as a peptide in the groove of a *class I MHC antigen*, or *class II MHC antigen*, molecule and, in addition to the interaction of the antigen-binding site with the peptide, *CD8* or *CD4*, which are associated with the T cell receptor, bind respectively to the conserved *domain* of the class I or class II molecule on the *antigen-presenting cell*. See Figures I2 and T1.

antigen excess Presence in a mixture of *antibody* and *antigen* of an amount of antigen sufficient to combine with all of the *antigen-binding sites* of the antibody molecules in the mixture and still leave free, uncombined, *epitopes* (i.e. antigenic determinants). Thus, *soluble complexes* are formed. A phenomenon explained by the *lattice hypothesis*. Soluble antigen–antibody complexes formed *in vivo* in conditions of antigen excess are of considerable importance in immunopathology as such complexes give rise to *Arthus*-type *reactions* when injected experimentally and are found in the lesions of *serum sickness, glomerulonephritis* and other *hypersensitivity* diseases. See also *antibody excess*.

antigen gain The acquisition by cells of new *epitopes* either not normally present or not normally accessible in the parent tissue. Often follows mutational change, e.g. in tumour cells, or lysogenic conversion in bacteria.

antigen presentation The presence on the surface of a cell of *antigen* in a form that allows its recognition by the T cell receptor (*TCR*). This usually requires that the antigen be presented as a small peptide in the groove of a syngeneic *major histocompatibility complex* (MHC) antigen molecule. Thus most nucleated cells can present antigen (of intracellular origin) on *class I MHC antigen* molecules. Professional *antigen-presenting cells* are *class II MHC antigen*+ and present antigen (from extracellular sources) on class II molecules. Antigen presentation usually requires prior *antigen processing* to provide suitable peptides for binding to the MHC molecules. *Superantigens* bind to MHC molecules but not in the groove and not in an *MHC restricted* fashion. See Figures A2 and A3.

antigen-presenting cell Cell that carries antigenic peptides bound to its own *major histocompatibility complex* (MHC) molecules in such a way that the peptide–MHC complex can be recognized by the T cell receptor (*TCR*). Recognition of this complex usually results in induction of an *immune response*. Such induction is *MHC restricted*, so the antigen-presenting cell and the antigen-recognizing *lymphocyte* must be *syngeneic*. See also *accessory cell*.

antigen processing The intracellular mechanism by which protein *antigens* are broken down to form small peptides which, on binding to *major histocompatibility complex* (MHC) molecules, can be presented (see *antigen presentation*) to the *TCR* (T cell receptor). The pathways of antigen processing are different for peptides that bind to *class I MHC antigens* or to *class*

II MHC antigens. (a) Class I MHC antigens bind antigenic peptides from *intracellular* sources (e.g. from proteins derived from viral genes incorporated into the host genome of a cell). Following their formation, these intracellular proteins are cleaved into peptides in the cytoplasm possibly by *proteasomes.* Peptides of around nine residues are then transported by *TAP* proteins across the membrane into the *endoplasmic reticulum* which contains newly synthesized class I MHC molecules. The peptides bind to, and stabilize the structure of, these molecules. The resulting class I MHC-peptide complex is transported to the Golgi system and thence out to the plasma membrane for antigen presentation. See Figure A2. (b) Class II MHC antigens bind antigenic peptides from *extracellular* sources. Proteins are endocytosed and degraded to peptides in specialized endosomal compartments, found in *antigen-presenting cells*. Since class II MHC antigen in the endoplasmic reticulum is linked to *invariant chain* (q.v.), it is unable to bind to intracellularly derived peptides found there. However, class II MHC is transported to the peptide-rich endosomal compartment, and there the invariant chain is degraded, freeing the class II molecule to bind to the exogenously derived peptide. The class II-peptide complex is then transported to the cell surface for antigen presentation. See Figure A3.

antigenic competition Phenomenon seen following *challenge* with an *antigen* in an animal responding to a different antigen. The animal fails to respond, or shows a diminished response, to the second antigen.

antigenic deletion Loss or masking of *epitopes* from cells whose parent tissue normally carries them. May result from neoplastic or other mutational change in the parent tissue and may be due to loss or repression of genetic material from the cell.

antigenic determinant Synonym for *epitope* q.v.

antigenic drift Slow *antigenic variation* over time in the *protective antigens* of a

pathogen such that the host's *immunity*, stemming from previous encounters with the organism, is partially overcome leading to minor illness. Especially noticeable in the case of the influenza A virus.

antigenic modulation See *modulation.*

antigenic profile The overall antigenic structure and arrangement of a cell or tissue.

antigenic reversion Antigenic change in adult cells such that the *antigenic profile* reverts from the adult form to a form existing in immature or fetal cells. Such reversion may follow neoplastic change.

antigenic shift A sudden, major, *antigenic variation* in the *protective antigens* of a pathogen such that any *immunity*, stemming from previous exposure to the organism, that the host may possess is totally overcome. Especially associated with the influenza A virus where it leads to worldwide epidemics.

antigenic variation There are two types: (1) A means by which certain parasites, especially trypanosomes, plasmodia and *Borrelia*, are enabled to survive the *immune response* of their host. When this response destroys the bulk of the parasite population a few survive. These survivors possess a cell surface of entirely different *antigenic* composition from that of their parents and grow into a second large parasitic population. This in turn is eliminated except for a few organisms of a third antigenic type. The cycle may be repeated many times: amongst the trypanosomes, over one hundred sequential types with no repetitions have been recorded. This type of variation is due to the expression of a new gene from a pre-existing set of *isotypes* of the antigen. (2) A phenomenon especially associated with the influenza virus which, unlike many viruses, undergoes spontaneous antigenic variation both as a slow *antigenic drift* from year to year and the occasional sudden emergence of a strain with new major

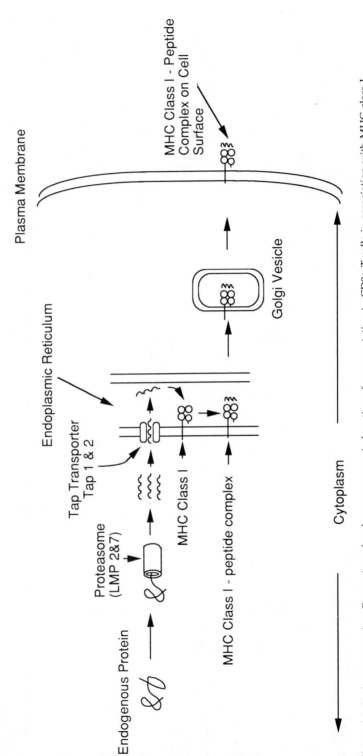

Figure A2. Antigen processing. Processing of endogenous, e.g. viral, antigen for presentation to CD8+ T cells in association with MHC class I.

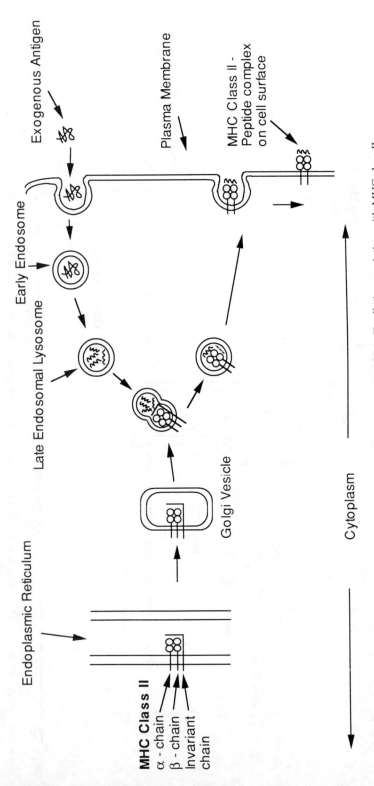

Figure A3. Antigen processing. Processing of exogenous antigen for presentation to CD4+ T cells in association with MHC class II.

antigens (*antigenic shift*). This type is the result of mutation.

antigenicity Capacity of a substance to act as an *antigen*. Term often also used synonymously with *immunogenicity* q.v.

antiglobulin test Originally a *haemagglutination test* in which the addition of anti *immunoglobulin* caused *agglutination* of red cells coated with non-agglutinating *antibody*: thus demonstrating that the anti red cell antibody had reacted with the cells. For example, human red cells are not agglutinated by *IgG* antibody bound to them but, after washing to remove free immunoglobulin, they are agglutinated by addition of an antiserum to human IgG. The antiglobulin test principle is now extended to the detection of antibody bound to a wide range of surfaces. See Figure A4.

antinuclear antibody See *anti nuclear antibody*.

antiserum *Serum* from any animal, which contains *antibodies* against a stated antigen, e.g. anti *ovalbumin*.

antitoxin *Antibody* against a bacterial toxin (usually *exotoxin*) or an *antiserum* containing such antibody.

antivenom See *anti venom*.

APAAP (alkaline phosphatase/anti alkaline phosphatase staining) A staining method for detecting *antigen* in cell preparations or tissue sections using a pre-formed complex of alkaline phosphatase with anti alkaline phosphatase. The cells or tissue section are incubated with a *primary antibody* specific for the antigen to be detected. This is followed by an excess of a *secondary antibody* against *IgG* and then by mouse anti alkaline phosphatase already bound to its antigen, alkaline phosphatase. The anti IgG cross-links the antigen-bound primary antibody to the APAAP complexes, which are then stained by incubation with a substrate (usually fast red or fast blue) to produce an insoluble, coloured product at the site of the antigen. The APAAP complex produces a multiplication effect due to the large number of enzyme molecules able to bind to the antigen, resulting in much greater sensitivity than a more direct antibody staining method. The principle is identical to the *peroxidase–anti-peroxidase technique* (PAP), see Figure P1.

APC See *antigen-presenting cell*.

Apo-1 The human equivalent of Fas. See *Fas*.

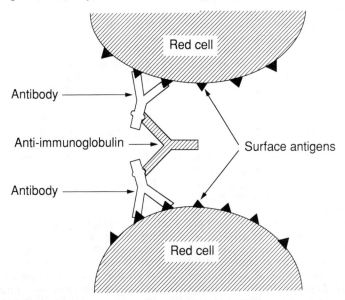

Figure A4. Antiglobulin test.

apoptosis Non-necrotic cell death in which cells shrink, show blebbing (zeiosis) with release of cell fragments, rounding-up of cell organelles and nucleus, and condensation of chromatin to give a sharp rim round the periphery of the nucleus. The DNA is cleaved by an endonuclease into equal-sized fragments. Apoptotic cells may not show impairment of membrane permeability, and death is not accompanied by release of cell contents as in necrosis. *Macrophages* are capable of removing large numbers of apoptotic cells without trace and this is probably an important disposal mechanism for senescent *neutrophil leucocytes*. Important mechanism for selection in maturation of both *T cells* and *B cells*; also the targets of *cytotoxic T lymphocytes* typically die by apoptosis. Of wide interest in development, both in immunology and elsewhere. Frequently, but not invariably, the form taken by *programmed cell death*.

ARC See *AIDS-related complex.*

ARDS See *acute respiratory distress syndrome.*

Arthus reaction An inflammatory reaction, characterized by oedema, haemorrhage and necrosis, that follows the administration of *antigen* to an animal that already possesses precipitating *antibody* to that antigen. Classically seen as an ulcer appearing some hours after intradermal injection of antigen into a *primed* animal, i.e. later than an *immediate hypersensitivity* reaction but earlier than a reaction of *cell-mediated immunity*. Caused by the formation, in the presence of *complement*, of *immune complexes* which adhere to the vascular endothelium, and become surrounded by fibrin, platelets and *neutrophil leucocytes*. The vessels become plugged with thrombi and there is exudation of fluid rich in neutrophils into the surrounding tissues. The term Arthus-type reaction has been applied to many hypersensitivity states in which the lesion is initiated by immune complexes as described in the original experiments of Arthus (see also *type III hypersensitivity reaction*). It is important in many clinical states, see *serum sickness, glomerulonephritis, farmer's lung.*

artificially acquired immunity *Protective immunity* acquired by *vaccination* or by *passive immunization*, in contrast to *naturally acquired immunity* which follows random contact with environmental antigens and organisms.

association constant A measure of the extent of a reversible association between two molecular species at equilibrium. For a reaction in which n molecules of substance A combine reversibly with m molecules of substance B, i.e. $n\mathrm{A} + m\mathrm{B} \leftrightarrow \mathrm{A_nB_m}$, the association constant is $[\mathrm{A_nB_m}]/[\mathrm{A}]^n[\mathrm{B}]^m$ where the symbols in brackets denote the molar concentrations (strictly, activities) at equilibrium. The dissociation constant is the reciprocal of the association constant.

asthma A common inflammatory lung disease characterized by general, but reversible, bronchial airway obstruction. Patients present with difficulty in breathing and wheeze due to the increased resistance to the passage of expired air. Sometimes a non-productive cough or shortness of breath on exercise are the only presenting features. Up to 20% of school children are affected and the incidence is increasing worldwide for no clear reason. The disease can be severe and asthmatics die each year in the UK. The airways have an inflammatory infiltrate of *lymphocytes* and *eosinophil leucocytes*, with smooth muscle hyperplasia, increased numbers of goblet cells and secretion of mucus, basement membrane thickening and collagen deposition. The smooth muscle becomes hyperreactive to contraction by *histamine*. Most acute cases are due to *IgE* mediated *immediate hypersensitivity (type I hypersensitivity reaction)* to inhaled *antigens (allergens)*.

ataxia telangiectasia Autosomal recessive *immunodeficiency* syndrome in children with *thymic hypoplasia* and *T cell* and *B cell* deficiencies. Associated with cerebellar ataxia, progressive dementia and oculocutaneous telangiectasia (dilation of capillaries). Defects of DNA repair cause multiple breaks in chromosomes at the site of *immunoglobulin genes* and *TCR genes*. High incidence of *lymphoma*.

atopic Adjectival form of *atopy* q.v.

atopic hypersensitivity See *atopy*.

atopy A constitutional or hereditary tendency to produce *IgE* antibody to common inhalant *allergens*, e.g. house dust mite (*Dermatophagoides pteronyssinus*) and grass pollen that provoke no *immune responses* in normal subjects.

attenuated vaccine A *live vaccine* containing organisms or viruses that have been cultured or otherwise treated under conditions in which they lose virulence but retain the capacity to stimulate a protective immune response (see *protective immunity*). Examples used in man include *BCG* and oral *poliomyelitis vaccine* (Sabin).

ATxBM mouse/rat (adult thymectomy: bone marrow reconstituted) Mouse or rat that has been deprived of *T lymphocytes* by whole body irradiation plus *thymectomy* followed by replacement of haemopoietic cells with an inoculation of T cell depleted *bone marrow* cells. Therefore it develops *B lymphocytes* but shows no responses of *cell-mediated immunity* and the only substances against which it can produce a humoral immune response (see *humoral immunity*) are *thymus independent antigens*. See also *nude mice*.

autoantibody *Antibody* capable of specific reaction with an *antigen* that is a normal constituent of the body of the individual in whom that antibody was formed. *In vitro* such antibodies are detected by their reaction with similar antigens, often obtained from another species.

autoantigen (self antigen) An *antigen* that is a normal constituent of the body and against which an *immune response* may be mounted by the same individual; this sometimes results in *autoimmune disease*.

autochthonous Derived from self. Syn. *autologous*.

autofluorescence Fluorescence of tissues due to molecules naturally present in them, i.e. unrelated to treatment of the tissue with *fluorochromes*.

autograft (syngeneic graft) Graft originated from, and applied to, the same individual, e.g. skin graft from back used for the repair of a facial burn. See also *transplantation terminology*.

autoimmune disease (1) Clinical disorder resulting from an *immune response* against *autoantigen*. To fit this definition precisely a disease should (a) show evidence of an immune response against autoantigen; (b) show lesions, with the presence of *immunologically competent* cells or *antibody*, related to the distribution of such antigens, and (c) be reproducible in experimental animals following injection of the relevant antigen, and be transferable from such animals to normal animals by *passive transfer* of *lymphocytes* or antibody. (2) The term is also used loosely of diseases associated with the presence of autoantibodies even when these are not of known significance in the pathogenesis.

autoimmunity Specific *humoral immunity* (*autoantibody* mediated) or *cell-mediated immunity* to constituents of the body's own tissues (*autoantigens*). If reactions between autoantibody or *T lymphocytes* and autoantigen result in tissue damage they may be regarded as *hypersensitivity* reactions. When such damage is sufficient to cause any clinical abnormality, an *autoimmune disease* is present.

autologous Derived from self; used of grafts, *antigens*, etc.

autoradiography Technique used to detect the presence of radioisotopes in cells and tissue sections, or in molecules (proteins, nucleic acids, etc.) that have been separated by electrophoresis, etc. The microscope slide, electrophoresis gel, etc. is covered with a photographic emulsion or film and exposed in the dark, usually for several days. When the photographic emulsion or film is developed the position of the radioisotope can be detected by the presence of silver grains. These may be seen as individual grains under the microscope or as blackened areas of film by the naked eye. Has also been adapted for use with sections prepared for electron microscopy. Alternatively, *antigens* may be detected by overlay with radiolabelled *antibody* followed by autoradiography. See also *fluorography*.

autoreactive lymphocytotoxic antibody *Autoantibodies* detected in *histocompatibility testing* that recognize common cell surface *antigens* of *lymphocytes* from random donors as well as those of *autologous* lymphocytes. They are almost always *antibodies* of *IgM* class and may not be detrimental to transplant function.

autosensitization Priming by *autoantigens*.

avidity An expression used to describe the strength of binding between macromolecules such as *antibody* and a complex *antigen*. Because the antigen has a range of *epitopes*, many of them different from each other, avidity is a composite description of the overall antibody–antigen interaction; it is, however, somewhat more complicated than a simple summation of affinities for individual epitopes since, because of the effective multivalency of the antigen there is often a cooperative 'bonus' effect. The avidity is often represented by the constant K_a, which is the value of the association constant for the reaction Ab + Ag = AbAg and which is obtained by assuming that this reaction roughly obeys the law of mass action. Avidity is, therefore, a function of the techniques used in its measurement and can only be expressed in arbitrary units.

axenic Adjective describing animals (i.e. protozoa upwards) reared in isolation from all other organisms. The absence of bacteria and larger organisms is relatively easily achieved; freedom from viruses much more difficult, especially as the latter may be incorporated in the genome. Cf. *gnotobiotic, germ free*.

azurophil granule Lysosome-like granule of the *neutrophil leucocyte*. Also known as primary granule as it first appears at the myeloblast stage, i.e. early in development (do not confuse with *primary lysosome* q.v.). Derived from the Golgi apparatus and contains acid hydrolases, cationic peptides and myeloperoxidase. Larger and denser than *specific granule* q.v.

B

B Alternative complement pathway component: see *Factor B*.

B cell See *B lymphocyte*; the two names are interchangeable.

B-1 lymphocyte A subset of *B lymphocytes* which appears early in ontogeny, is the major B cell type in infancy, and is then replaced by *conventional B lymphocytes*. Two populations: B-1a which express *CD5*; and B-1b which do not, have been reported. CD5+ B-1 cells are important in *autoimmune disease* since many *autoantibodies* are made by these cells. They are the commonest form of neoplastic B cell in *chronic lymphocytic leukaemia*.

B lymphocyte (also called a B cell; the two names are interchangeable) A *lymphocyte* that is derived from a precursor in the *bone marrow*, unlike the *T lymphocyte* which develops in the *thymus*. B lymphocytes are the mediators of *humoral immunity* and on stimulation by *antigen* they differentiate into *antibody*-forming *plasma cells* and B memory cells (see *immunological memory*). In the case of *thymus dependent antigens* this process requires cooperation with T lymphocytes (cf. *thymus independent antigens*). In birds, B lymphocyte maturation is determined by the *bursa of Fabricius*.

B lymphocyte receptor (B lymphocyte antigen receptor, B cell receptor) Synonym for *membrane immunoglobulin* (mIg), the transmembrane *antigen*-recognizing unit of the *B lymphocyte*.

B lymphocyte repertoire The number of different V_H region–V_L region combinations (i.e. *antigen-binding sites*) that the immune system is potentially capable of producing. This is considerably larger than the number of different *B lymphocyte receptors* present on the *B cells* of an individual at a given time.

B mouse See *ATxBM mouse/rat*.

bacille Calmette–Guérin See *BCG*.

bacterial agglutination The *agglutination* of bacteria by *antibody*. Tests based on this are widely used in diagnostic bacteriology either for the detection of antibody (e.g. Widal reaction) or for the identification of organisms isolated from clinical cases. The *in vivo* agglutination of bacteria may also play a part in their *immune elimination*.

bacteriolysis The destruction of bacteria by rupture so that the cells release their contents. The *membrane attack complex* of *complement* is bacteriolytic. Following *phagocytosis* and intracellular killing, bacteria are lysed by the digestive enzymes of phagocytic cells.

bacteriophage neutralization test See *phage neutralization test*.

BALT Bronchus-associated *lymphoid tissue*.

bare lymphocyte syndrome An autosomal recessive form of *SCID* in which there is a deficiency of *class II MHC antigen* gene expression. The cells of the immune system express few or no HLA-DP, -DQ or HLA-DR antigens (see *HLA histocompatibility system*) and there is therefore a defect of *antigen presentation* to *CD4+ T cells*, *immunodeficiency*, and an increased susceptibility to infection.

basement membrane antibody *Antibody* against *antigens* present in glomerular (GBM) and alveolar basement membranes causing acute *glomerulonephritis* (anti-GBM disease) which may be associated with lung haemorrhage (*Goodpasture's syndrome*).

basophil degranulation test An *in vitro* test for *immediate hypersensitivity*. The suspect *allergen* (*antigen*) is added to a *buffy coat* preparation from the patient believed to be *sensitized*. If *IgE* specific for the allergen is present on *basophil leucocytes* in the buffy coat they degranulate. Degranulation causes the basophils to lose their staining characteristics with toludine blue. Alternatively, the *histamine* released from the basophils as a proportion of total histamine can be measured to quantify the extent of degranulation.

basophil leucocyte A *leucocyte* derived from *bone marrow* and found in small numbers (less than 1%) in blood, which contains round granules of different sizes giving a basophilic reaction with normal stains. The granules contain heparin, also *histamine* and other *vascular permeability factors* that may be released at sites of inflammation or in *immediate hypersensitivity* reactions. Basophil leucocytes possess high affinity *Fc receptors* for *IgE* (FcεRI, see *Fcε receptors*). Cf. *mast cell*, which the basophil closely resembles.

B/B rat *Inbred strain* of rat which shows high incidence of spontaneous autoimmune diabetes (see *autoimmunity*) secondary to inflammation of the pancreatic islets of Langerhans, resulting in selective destruction of the insulin-producing β cells.

BCG Bacille Calmette–Guérin. A living attenuated bovine strain of *Mycobacterium tuberculosis* used as a vaccine to protect against tuberculosis (and leprosy). Prepared by two French workers, hence name.

bcl-2 Oncogene whose protein product (bcl-2) allows survival of cells which would otherwise die by *apoptosis* when deprived of appropriate growth factors or *cytokines*. If the cell expresses bcl-2 it can survive in the absence of such factors. Important in the development of *stem cells* in *bone marrow*, the *positive selection* of B cells of *germinal centres*,

inter alia. The *bcl*-2 gene family contains other members that regulate cell death, e.g. homodimers of the protein bax induce death, but bcl-2/bax heterodimers have no effect.

beige mouse An *inbred strain* of mouse that has a congenital defect in *lysosome* function, producing abnormalities in the function of several *leucocyte* populations. In particular, beige mice are partially (but not completely) deficient in *NK cells*, and show immune defects similar to *Chediak–Higashi syndrome* in man.

Bence–Jones protein Protein in urine of patients with *myelomatosis*. Precipitated by heating to 60°C but redissolves on further heating to 90°C. MW 46 kD. Consists of dimerized *light chains* of *myeloma protein*.

benign monoclonal gammopathy A *paraproteinaemia* characterized by the typical serum abnormality of this group of diseases, i.e. an electrophoretic spike of *myeloma protein*-type *immunoglobulin*, but without any of the other abnormalities associated with *myelomatosis*. Patients remain well and the prognosis is good.

berylliosis Disease caused by inhalation contact with beryllium mainly in industry. Persons who inhale dust containing compounds of beryllium may develop an acute chemical pneumonia or a more chronic pulmonary granulomatous disease (see *granuloma*) similar to sarcoidosis with *epithelioid cell* granulomata leading to pulmonary fibrosis. May also affect *lymph nodes*, skin, other tissues. Poorly understood but may involve *delayed-type hypersensitivity* to complexes of beryllium with macromolecules.

β (beta) **thromboglobulin** See Table C2.

β$_2$ microglobulin Protein (11 kD) structurally similar to a single immunoglobulin *constant region* which is found in free form in solution in biological fluids (in elevated levels in *AIDS*), but whose major importance is that it is normally linked non-covalently to the *class I*

MHC antigen molecule and stabilizes that molecule in the correct conformation for *antigen presentation*. Also associates with *CD1*.

BGG Bovine *gamma globulin*; commonly used as an *antigen* in experimental work.

bi-specific antibody molecule See *bispecific antibody molecule*.

binding constant See *association constant*.

binding site Term used of *antigen-binding site* and other specified sites of attachment of macromolecules to one another.

biochemical sequestration Inability of *hidden determinants* on a molecule or cell to stimulate an *immune response* or to combine with *antibody*. Following a structural change in the molecule or cell such determinants may be revealed and become capable of recognition. Such changes in *autoantigens* may result in *autoantibody* production. See *rheumatoid factor*.

biotin/avidin/streptavidin system A technique for the detection of *antigen* or *antibody* in tissues, on a synthetic membrane (e.g. in *immunoblotting*) or on plastic as in *ELISA* assays. In its simplest form, a biotinylated antibody (i.e. bonded to the vitamin biotin) is bound to the antigen under investigation. The resulting immune complexes are then detected using labelled avidin or streptavidin (avidin is an egg white protein that binds strongly to biotin; the label can be a radioisotope, *fluorochrome*, gold particle or an enzyme). In variations of this system: (a) the *primary antibody* is overlaid with biotinylated anti-*immunoglobulin* followed by labelled avidin or streptavidin; (b) unlabelled avidin or streptavidin is used to cross link the biotinylated anti-immunoglobulin to biotinylated enzyme (horseradish peroxidase or alkaline phosphatase). This is called the 'bridge' method; and (c) a complex of avidin or streptavidin and biotinylated enzyme is allowed to bind to the biotinylated anti

immunoglobulin. This resembles the *peroxidase–anti peroxidase* (PAP) *technique* (see Figure P1). Avidin and streptavidin have four binding sites for biotin, giving a multiplication effect. These sites have a very high affinity for biotin allowing detection of very low concentrations of antigen. Streptavidin is frequently used in preference to avidin as it is said to give lower backgrounds.

bird fancier's lung Restrictive lung disease (a syndrome of *extrinsic allergic alveolitis*, q.v.) caused by exposure to dust containing *antigens* derived from the blood *plasma* of birds, especially albumin and *gamma globulin*. These are present in bird faeces and also in 'bloom' (dust) from the skin and feathers. The disease is characterized by attacks of breathlessness with fever due predominantly to a *hypersensitivity* reaction. In the acute phase this has the timing of an *Arthus reaction* (*type III hypersensitivity reaction*) in the lung (4–8 hours post antigen exposure) and is characterized by a transient *neutrophil leucocyte* infiltrate into the lung interstitium. This soon evolves into a *lymphocyte* infiltrate, predominantly of *CD8+ T cells* which characterize prolonged exposure or chronic disease. Patients' sera characteristically have raised *IgG* levels and high titres of *antibody* to bird *serum* proteins. Cross reactivity between avian species is enough to allow one antigen source, e.g. pigeon serum, to be used in tests for exposure to other birds.

bispecific antibody molecule *Antibody* molecule with one *antigen-binding site* specific for one *antigen*, and the other antigen-binding site specific for another. A deliberately engineered laboratory artefact, following recombination of *heavy chains* and *light chains* derived from two different specific antibodies.

blast cell A cell, usually large (diameter >8 μm), with ill-differentiated cytoplasm rich in RNA and actively synthesizing DNA (as shown by the rapid incorporation of tritiated thymidine). The nuclear patterns of blast cells vary and help to determine morphologically the series to which it belongs, e.g. *plasmablast*, myeloblast (of *myeloid cell series*), etc.

blast transformation See *lymphocyte activation*.

blocking antibody (1) In *agglutination* tests; *antibody* that, because of low *valency* (e.g. *IgG*) or attachment to *epitopes* embedded in the surface, may coat cells and prevent their agglutination by high valency *IgM*. It may be detected by the *antiglobulin test*. (2) In *immediate hypersensitivity*; antibody of IgG type that may combine preferentially with *antigen* (or *allergen*) thus preventing it from reacting with *IgE*. Blocking antibody is thus able to inhibit immediate hypersensitivity reactions. In *hyposensitization*, an attempt is made to encourage preferential formation of blocking antibody in atopic (see *atopy*) persons by repeated injections of allergen.

blood group Classification of *isoantigens* on the surfaces of erythrocytes. The most important blood groups in man are those of the *ABO*, and *Rhesus blood group systems* q.v.

blood group substance Soluble substance present in body fluids that bears *blood group* specificity, i.e. shares *epitopes* with red cell surface *isoantigens* (see also *ABO blood group substances*).

bone marrow The soft tissue that fills the cavities of bones. Red marrow is actively haemopoietic (i.e. blood forming) and is found in developing bone, ribs, vertebrae and parts of long bones. It contains all the cells and corpuscles (with their precursors) of the circulating blood, and also megakaryocytes, reticulum cells, *macrophages* and *plasma cells*. It contains *lymphocyte* stem cells and is the principal site of formation of *B lymphocytes* and *pre-T lymphocytes* (but not mature *T lymphocytes*) in the adult. In adult animals much of the red marrow is replaced by fatty tissue and becomes yellow marrow.

booster dose A dose of *antigen* given after the *priming dose* to stimulate an accelerated *secondary immune response*. Especially used to refer to doses of *vaccine* given at intervals of a few months or years after a preliminary course of injections in an *immunization* programme.

bovine serum albumin *Albumin* from the *serum* of cattle, used as an experimental antigen.

Boyden chamber An apparatus used in tests for *chemotaxis*. Consists of two compartments separated by a microporous filter. Cells are placed in the upper compartment and the chemotactic agent in the lower. Cells sediment onto the filter and, if they are attracted by the agent, migrate through its pores. The filter is then stained and cell migration measured.

bradykinin A basic nonapeptide, one of the vasoactive plasma *kinins* q.v. whose action is slow compared with that of *histamine*. It is detectable in the tissues in experimental *anaphylaxis*, indicating that the kinin system probably plays a part in the pathogenesis of *immediate hypersensitivity* lesions.

Bruton type hypogammaglobulinaemia See *X-linked agammaglobulinaemia*.

BSA See *bovine serum albumin*.

buffy coat The layer of *white cells* that forms between the red cell layer and the *plasma* when unclotted blood is centrifuged.

Burkitt's lymphoma Malignant tumour of *B lymphocytes* affecting *lymphoid tissues* especially in the jaws and abdominal viscera. Common in, but not exclusive to, African children. Associated with hot, humid climate in circumscribed area of Africa corresponding to areas where disease-carrying mosquitoes are found. EB virus, a herpestype virus, has been isolated from the *lymphoma* cells and has also been shown to cause *infectious mononucleosis* (glandular fever). *Antibody* to EB virus is found in the sera of patients with Burkitt's lymphoma. The B cells carry *CD77* as a characteristic marker. CD77 is a marker for *germinal centre* B cells and Burkitt's lymphoma may represent a malignant variant of these. The disease tends to remit and to respond to chemotherapy. This may be related to an *immune response* against the tumour.

bursa of Fabricius A sac-like lymphoepithelial structure arising as a dorsal diverticulum from the cloaca of young birds. First described in 1621 by Hieronymus Fabricius, an Italian anatomist, it is composed entirely of plicae containing numerous *lymphoid follicles*. *B cell* lymphopoiesis takes place within these and continues until the structure involutes at about the time of sexual maturity. The bursa is associated with *humoral immunity*. *Bursectomized* chickens fail to make *antibodies* to a variety of *antigens* and *plasma cells* and *germinal centres* are reduced or absent in their *lymphoid tissues*.

bursectomy Removal or destruction of the avian *bursa of Fabricius*. When this is done surgically *in ovo* or shortly after hatching, or *in ovo* by administration of testosterone or other hormones, the development of *B lymphocytes* is prevented.

byssinosis Disease of workers in vegetable fibre industry, e.g. cotton, flax, jute, hemp. Presents with chest tightness after a period of absence from work. thus 'Monday morning fever' and 'return to work fever'. Suggested to be due to hypersensitivity to vegetable fibre dusts.

bystander lysis Non-specific lysis of tissue cells during an *immune response* against other, specific, target structures (see *bystander phenomena*).

bystander phenomena The non-specific effects (including lysis) of an *immune response* on tissues which are not themselves specific targets of that response, but which are susceptible to the action of non-specific factors released during the response.

C

C Symbol for *complement*.

C exon Gene coding for the *constant region* of an *immunoglobulin* molecule *heavy chain* or *light chain*. The heavy chain C exon is divided by *introns* into separate units corresponding to the *homology regions* of the heavy chain. See Figure I4.

C-gene See *C exon*.

c-Kit ligand (stem cell factor) A *cytokine* that binds to a membrane *receptor* on haemopoietic *stem cells*. It is made by and expressed on stromal cells of the *bone marrow* and contact with these stromal cells is required for stem cells to mature and to respond to other *colony stimulating factors*. The stem cell receptor is a *protein tyrosine kinase*.

C reactive protein Serum protein of the *pentraxin* family normally present in *serum* but increased in concentration in many inflammatory processes (see *acute phase reactants*). Synthesized by hepatocytes (liver cells) in response to *IL-1* and *IL-6*, and also by *macrophages* in inflammatory sites. Reacts with phosphorylcholine, and also binds to other choline phosphatides and to polyanions. Following binding to ligands, C reactive protein activates the *classical complement pathway* by binding to C1q (see *C1*). It can thus induce *opsonization*, e.g. of the bacterium to which it is bound.

C region See *constant region*.

C1 The first component of *complement*. Comprises three subcomponents C1q, C1r, C1s which occur as a macromolecular complex *in vivo* in the presence of Ca²⁺ ions. Heat labile. C1q carries the site which binds to the *Fc fragment* of *immune complexes* containing *IgG* and

IgM (in man). Following binding to complexes, C1r is converted to C̄1r which cleaves C1s to form C̄1s, C̄1s carries the enzymatic site which acts on *C4* and *C2* and results in their cleavage. Note: the overbar indicates that the component is activated.

C1 inhibitor (C1 esterase inhibitor or inactivator) An inhibitor of the activated esterase formed from *C1*. An α₂ globulin normally present in *serum*. Deficient in *hereditary angio-oedema*. Also inhibits the Hageman factor fragments, *kallikreins*, plasminogen activator, plasmin.

C1INH See *C1 inhibitor*.

C2 The second component of *complement*. Split by *C1*, and, in the presence of Mg²⁺ ions, complexes with C4b (see *C4*) to form the *C3 convertase* enzyme C4b2a. Heat labile.

C3 The third component of *complement*. Actually reacts fourth in the haemolytic *complement activation* sequence, thus EAC1423 (see *EAC*). Serum concentration much higher than that of other complement components (500–1000 µg/ml). Contains two polypeptide chains (α and β) linked by disulphide and non-covalent bonds. Both the classical complement pathway *C3 convertase* (C4b2a) and the *alternative pathway C3 convertase* (C3bBbP) split the α-chain to give a small fragment *C3a* and the remainder of the molecule is then known as *C3b*.

C3 convertase Enzymes of the *complement* system that will cleave *C3* into *C3a* and *C3b*. The classical complement pathway C3 convertase is the bi-molecular complex C4b2a. Distinguish this from *alternative pathway C3 convertase* which is a complex of *C3b*, Factor B and *properdin* (C3bBbP).

C3 nephritic factor An *autoantibody* with specificity for the *alternative pathway C3 convertase* C3bBbP. It stabilizes the convertase and renders it resistant to the decay dissociation effect of *Factor H*. Thus it causes intense activation of the alternative pathway. Found in the sera of a proportion of patients with hypocomplementaemic membranoproliferative glomerulonephritis (see *hypocomplementaemia* and *glomerulonephritis*).

C3a A biologically active fragment of *complement* component *C3*. It is a low molecular weight basic polypeptide (MW about 9 kD) split from the N-terminal end of the α chain of C3 by *C3 convertase* and other tryptic enzymes. C3a is biologically active as an *anaphylatoxin*. This activity is destroyed by *anaphylatoxin inactivator* a naturally occurring carboxypeptidase N which digests the C-terminal arginine from C3a.

C3b An active fragment of *complement* component *C3*. It is produced when the α chain of C3 is digested by *C3 convertase*, splitting off *C3a* q.v. This exposes a transient thiol ester group which can bind to ester or amide groups thus resulting in its covalent linkage to cell surfaces or *immune complexes*. It can also interact with water rendering the thiol ester group inactive. C3b has an affinity for cell surfaces, i.e. for the C3b receptors (*CR1*) present on *macrophages*, *neutrophil leucocytes*, *B lymphocytes* and possibly *T lymphocytes*, hence C3b enhances *immune adherence*, *phagocytosis* and acts as an *opsonin*. *Factor I* cleaves the α chain of C3b to form *iC3b*.

C3b inactivator See *Factor I*.

C3b receptors See *CR1* (CD35; binds *C3b* and *C4*b), *CR2* (CD21; binds C3d a cleavage product of C3b), *CR3* (CD11b; binds *iC3b*) and *CR4* (CD11c; binds iC3b).

C3bi Synonym for *iC3b*.

C3H mice One of the *inbred strains* of mice commonly used in immunological experiments. Many substrains exist some of which exhibit experimentally valuable mutations, e.g. lymphocytes of the C3H/HeJ substrain are unresponsive to *lipopolysaccharide*.

C4 The fourth component of *complement*. Actually reacts second in haemolytic *complement activation* sequence, thus EAC14 (see *EAC*). Second most abundant complement component. Substrate for *C1* which cleaves C4 by splitting it to produce an active part, C4b, and a fragment, C4a. See also *C2*. Destroyed by hydrazine and other primary amines. Heat stable. Consists of three polypeptide chains, α, β, γ. C4a has *anaphylatoxin* activity. C4b can bind to cell surfaces and *immune complexes* by a transiently expressed thiol ester bond which is inactivated by water.

C4 binding protein Serum control protein of the *complement* cascade (see *cascade reaction*). A heptamer made up of *short consensus repeat* units, it controls the activity of the *classical complement pathway* in two ways: (a) it acts as a cofactor to the enzyme *Factor I* in the cleavage of C4b (see *C4*) so that cleaved C4b can no longer form a functional *C3 convertase* and, (b) it accelerates the decay of the classical pathway C3 convertase by displacing *C2*.

C5 The fifth component of *complement*. On activation by *C5 convertase* C4b2aC3b, or by C3bBbP(C3b), the *alternative pathway* convertase, a small fragment, *C5a*, MW 7–12 kD is split off. This fragment acts as an *anaphylatoxin* and has chemotactic activity for *leucocytes* (see *chemotaxis*). The remainder of the split C5 molecule, C5b, forms a complex with *C6*, *C7*, *C8* and *C9* which forms the *membrane attack complex* and has an affinity for cell membranes and damages them. This mediates *immune cytolysis* and *haemolysis*.

C5 convertase An enzymic protein complex that allows the initiation of the *membrane attack complex* by cleavage of *C5* to C5a and C5b. This is the last enzymic step in the *complement* cascade. The classical and *alternative pathway* C5 convertases change their substrate specificity from *C3* to C5 on addition to each of an extra molecule of C3b (forming C4b2aC3b and C3bBbPC3b respectively).

C5a Peptide with activity as chemotactic factor (see *chemotaxis*) and *anaphylatoxin*. Derived from *C5* by tryptic cleavage by *C5 convertase*. In man, a 74 residue, glycosylated peptide. An *anaphylatoxin inactivator* with carboxypeptidase-N activity occurs naturally in human serum and removes the C-terminal arginine from C5a to form C5a$_{desArg}$. C5a$_{desArg}$ lacks anaphylatoxin activity, but retains some chemotactic activity. The C5a receptor (CD88) has been identified on *neutrophil leucocytes*. It is a *Type III transmembrane protein* of the *rhodopsin superfamily* with seven membrane spanning domains (see Figure T3).

C6 The sixth component of *complement*. A single polypeptide chain which forms part of the *membrane attack complex*. See also *C5*.

C7 The seventh component of *complement*. A single polypeptide chain which forms part of the *membrane attack complex*. See also *C5*.

C8 The eighth component of *complement*. Consists of three polypeptide chains, α, β, γ and forms part of the *membrane attack complex*.

C9 The final component of *complement*. When *C3–C9* have reacted in a haemolytic sequence, the red cell membrane is damaged by bound C5b–9, i.e. the *membrane attack complex* and the cell undergoes lysis. Although not absolutely essential for complement-mediated lysis, C9 speeds up the low grade lytic activity of the C5b–8 complex.

caecal tonsils See *tonsil*.

calcineurin A protein phosphatase which is involved in regulation of transcription of *cytokine* genes (e.g. for *IL-2*) in *T cells*. *Cyclophilins* and *FKBP*, once they have bound the drugs *cyclosporin A* and *FK506®* respectively, bind

to calcineurin and inhibit its action. This is believed to be the basis of the *immunosuppressive* action of these drugs.

C$_α$; C$_δ$; C$_ε$; C$_γ$; C$_κ$; C$_λ$; C$_μ$ The *constant regions* of the *immunoglobulin* chains corresponding to the appropriate subscript Greek letter. See Table I1.

capping Accumulation of clusters or patches of aggregated proteins at one site on the cell surface. Follows the aggregation of surface components of cell membranes, e.g. by the action of polyvalent ligands (see *patching*). When cells with such patches move, the latter are swept to the posterior area of the cell forming a cap there. Capping is an energy requiring process, cf. patching.

capsular polysaccharide Polysaccharides present as constituents of bacterial capsules. Often *antigenic* and are *TI-2 antigens*. The best studied are those of *Streptococcus pneumoniae* (pneumococcus) but many other organisms have polysaccharide capsules.

carbon clearance test A test used to measure the activity of the *mononuclear phagocyte* system in experimental animals. A suspension of colloidal carbon particles is inoculated intravenously and blood samples collected at short intervals thereafter. Disappearance of carbon from the blood with time is taken as a measure of removal by mononuclear phagocytes.

cardiolipin antibodies (anti-phospholipid antibodies) *Autoantibodies* to cell membrane phospholipid. They are found in several clinical conditions, i.e. recurrent thrombotic events, thrombocytopenia, recurrent abortions and connective tissue diseases such as systemic lupus erythematosus (*SLE*). The term anti-phospholipid syndrome is often used to describe conditions associated with the presence of these antibodies which are also detected in the *Wassermann test* for syphilis.

carrier Macromolecule to which a *hapten* is conjugated *in vitro*, or to which it may become attached *in vivo*, and which renders the hapten capable of stimulating an *immune response*. Note that the word 'carrier' in *heterologous carrier vaccines* is used with a somewhat different meaning.

carrier specificity Term used of *antibody* (or of a *cell-mediated immune* response) formed in response to injection of *hapten* conjugated to a *carrier* macromolecule, and which has specificity for the hapten–carrier complex but not for free hapten nor for hapten bound to an unrelated carrier.

cascade reaction A sequential reaction in which each event initiates the next event in the sequence. Used of enzymic reactions such as *complement activation*, blood coagulation, etc.

CBA mouse An *inbred strain* of mouse. Many substrains exist of which CBA/H-T6, which is homozygous for the cytological marker translocation T6, is the most important to the immunologist. See *T6 marker*.

CCP superfamily (complement control protein superfamily) See *SCR superfamily*.

CD antigens A classification of cell surface proteins as 'clusters of differentiation' *antigens* based on their reactions with panels of *monoclonal antibodies*. The CD numbers are assigned to molecules by agreement at international workshops. The CD nomenclature has gained general acceptance as a convenient way of listing cell surface molecules. Cell surface proteins that are still in process of allocation to a CD are given a provisional identity by the addition of 'w' (workshop) to the likely number, e.g. CDw90 for the *Thy 1 antigen* at the time of writing. The prefixed abbreviation 'a' (rarely 'α') is used to mean 'anti' as in 'aCD3' (*antibody* to *CD3*). Table C1 lists all of the presently identified CD antigens, some of these are given more extensive descriptions below. Figure C3 shows a selection of CD antigens on the cell membrane.

CD1 A *Type I transmembrane protein* of the *Ig superfamily*. Resembles *class I*

MHC antigens and the molecule is normally associated non-covalently with β_2 *microglobulin*. However CD1 does not show polymorphism. There are several CD1 genes and in man CD1a, b, c and d are expressed on the cell surface. CD1 is found on cortical *thymocytes* (see *thymus*) but not on *T cells*. It is also found on *dendritic cells*. A function in *antigen presentation* has been suggested.

CD2 (LFA-2) A *Type I transmembrane protein* of the *Ig superfamily* with one extracellular V-like and one C-like domain. In man, a *T cell* marker, but also found on *NK cells*, and is the E-rosette receptor (see *E-rosette forming cell*). It is an adhesion molecule whose ligand is *LFA-3* (CD58) found on many cells. Thus it may play a role as a *costimulatory molecule* in T cell clustering with *accessory cells* in the response to *antigen*, in T cell signalling and also in binding of *cytotoxic T lymphocytes* to their targets. See Figure C3.

CD3 A multichain molecule comprising *Ig superfamily* γ, δ, and ε chains associated with ζ (zeta) *chains* and η (eta) *chains* either as ζ homodimers or as ζ–η heterodimers. All are *Type I transmembrane proteins*. CD3 is always associated with the T cell receptor (*TCR*) (α and β chains, or γ and δ chains) to make up a seven-chain complex. The TCR–CD3 complex is the defining feature of the *T lymphocyte*. CD3 and the associated η and ζ chains are involved in signalling on contact of the TCR with *major histocompatibility complex*-associated *antigen*. See Figure T1.

CD4 A *Type I transmembrane protein* of the *Ig superfamily*, CD4 has four *immunoglobulin*-like extracellular domains. It is found on a high proportion of mature *T lymphocytes* (60% in human blood) and these are always *CD8* negative. When T cells recognize *major histocompatibility complex* (MHC) class II-associated antigen, CD4 binds as an accessory molecule to the *class II MHC antigen* molecule on the *antigen-presenting* cell. The CD4+ phenotype is associated with *helper T lymphocyte* function though the association is not absolute. CD4 may act as a signalling molecule since the cytoplasmic domain contains both serine/threonine and tyrosine phosphorylation sites. CD4 acts as the *receptor* for *HIV* which progressively destroys CD4+ *lymphocytes*. Human *monocytes* and *macrophages* also express CD4 and thus may also become infected with HIV. CD4 is found on *thymocytes* which early in development (in the cortex of the *thymus*) are CD4+CD8+ and later (in the medulla of the thymus) either CD4+CD8– or CD4–CD8+. See Figures C1, C3 and T3.

CD5 A *Type I transmembrane protein* of the *scavenger receptor superfamily*. Present on *thymocytes* and on all mature *T lymphocytes*. Binds to CD72 on *B lymphocytes*. Absent from most B cells in normal blood but is found on a subset (B-1a lymphocytes, see *B-1 lymphocyte*) which makes many *autoantibodies* and may be important in *autoimmune diseases*. In most cases of *chronic lymphocytic leukaemia* the neoplastic B cells are CD5 positive.

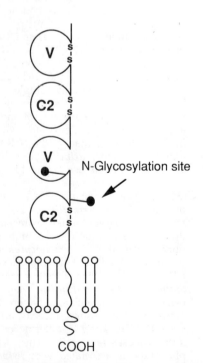

N-Glycosylation site

COOH

Figure C1. CD4.

CD8 A heterodimer consisting of an α and a β chain, both *Type I transmembrane proteins* of the *Ig superfamily*. It is found on *thymocytes* (see *CD4*) and on a minor population (15–25%) of mature *T lymphocytes* and these are always CD4 negative. Also present on some *NK cells*. When T lymphocytes recognize *major histocompatibility complex* (MHC) class I-associated antigens (see *class I MHC antigens*), CD8 binds as an accessory molecule to the class I molecule on the *antigen-presenting cell*. The CD8+ phenotype is associated with *cytotoxic T lymphocyte* function though the association is not absolute. See Figure C2.

CD10 A *Type II transmembrane protein* with activity as a neutral endopeptidase. Formerly known as CALLA (common acute lymphoblastic leukaemia antigen) since it is present on *B lymphocyte* and *T lymphocyte* precursors and is used as a marker for *acute lymphoblastic leukaemia*. It is also present on various other cells including *neutrophil leucocytes*.

CD11a, b and c Members of the *integrin superfamily* (*Type I transmembrane proteins*) which are the α chains of leucocyte integrins and each of which forms a heterodimer with the β_2 integrin chain, to make three integrins, viz. CD11a/CD18, CD11b/CD18, and CD11c/CD18. See *CD18*.

(a) **CD11a/CD18** (LFA-1) ($\alpha_L\beta_2$) is found on all *leucocytes* and binds to *ICAMs-1*, *-2*, and *-3*. See Figures C3 and I7.

(b) **CD11b/CD18** (MAC-1; Mo-1) (CR3) ($\alpha_M\beta_2$) is found on cells of the *myeloid cell series* (*neutrophil leucocytes, monocytes, macrophages*) and on *NK cells*. Binds to ICAM-1 and to the complement protein *iC3b*.

(c) **CD11c/CD18** (p150,95) (CR4) ($\alpha_X\beta_2$) is found on myeloid cells and on *dendritic cells*. It is a marker for hairy cell leukaemia. Binding characteristics not fully studied but it binds to iC3b.

These are important adhesion molecules for attachment to vascular endothelium and for cell–cell clustering. LFA-1 (CD11a/CD18) is upregulated on *T lymphocytes* on activation with anti-

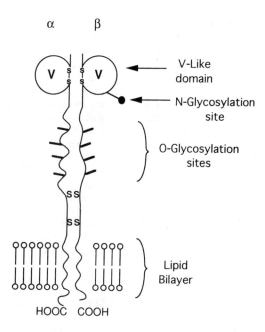

α   β

V-Like domain

N-Glycosylation site

O-Glycosylation sites

Lipid Bilayer

HOOC COOH

Figure C2. CD8.

gen; CD11b/CD18 and CD11c/CD18 are upregulated on myeloid cells by inflammatory mediators, e.g. chemotactic factors (see *chemotaxis*).

CD14 A *GPI anchor*-linked glycoprotein frequently used as a marker for *monocytes* and *macrophages*, though it may be found on other cell types. On mononuclear phagocytes (see *mononuclear phagocyte* system) it binds the complex of *lipopolysaccharide* (LPS) with *LPS binding protein*, thus allowing LPS to activate monocytes to produce TNF-α and other *cytokines*.

CD15 The Lewis x (Le x) *blood group* pentasaccharide which is recognized in its sialylated form (CD15s) by E-selectin and P-selectin (see *selectins*). It may itself be a component of glycolipids and membrane glycoproteins. Present on *neutrophil leucocytes, eosinophil leucocytes* and *monocytes* and is an important ligand for the selectin-mediated adhesion of these cells to vascular endothelium.

CD16 (FcγRIII) See *Fcγ receptor*.

CD18 *Type I transmembrane glycoprotein* of the *integrin superfamily* and

is the β$_2$ chain of that family. Associates with *CD11a, b, and c* (q.v.) to form *leucocyte*-specific heterodimers, see Figure I7. The α chains (CD11) contain the *ligand* binding site which is regulated by CD18. Mg^{2+} ions are essential for function. Defects in the gene for CD18 are associated with *leucocyte adhesion deficiency* (LAD) q.v., a severe immunodeficiency syndrome.

CD19 A *Type I transmembrane protein* of the *Ig superfamily*. Present on *B lymphocytes* but not *plasma cells* and is frequently used as a phenotypic marker for B cells. Probably plays a role, in association with other cell-surface molecules, in signal transduction in B cells.

CD20 A *Type III transmembrane protein* with four membrane-spanning regions. A specific marker for *B lymphocytes* in which it may function as a calcium channel.

CD21 See *CR2*.

CD22 A *Type I transmembrane protein* of the *Ig superfamily*. Found in two forms, α with five *immunoglobulin*-like domains and β with seven. Present on many *B lymphocytes*, but lost after the B cells are activated. CD22 may contribute to B cell–T cell adhesion and may bind to *CD45*.

CD23 (FcεRII) A *Type II transmembrane protein* containing a C-type *lectin* domain. Found on *B lymphocytes* very early after activation, e.g. by *IL-4*. Also present on *follicular dendritic cells* (FDC) which release soluble CD23. It is a low affinity IgE *Fc receptor*, and performs this function on *macrophages* and *eosinophil leucocytes* as well as on B cells. B cell CD23 also binds to *CD21* (CR2) on *T lymphocytes*.

CD25 (IL-2Rα) The alpha chain of the *IL-2 receptor* (q.v.).

CD28 A *Type I transmembrane protein* disulphide-linked homodimer and member of the *Ig superfamily*. Found on *thymocytes* and on most peripheral *T lymphocytes* and expression is increased when T cells are activated. CD28 binds to a *B lymphocyte*-specific protein *CD80* (B7/BB1). This binding is believed to contribute an important costimulatory signal in *T cell* interactions with *B cells* or other CD80+ *accessory cells*.

CD29 The β₁ integrin chain. See *CD49* and *integrin superfamily*.

CD31 (PECAM-1) A *Type I transmembrane protein* of the *Ig superfamily* with six *immunoglobulin*-like domains. Present on many *leucocytes* and its presence on *T lymphocytes* is correlated with the presence of CD45RA (see *CD45*). Also found on vascular endothelial cells and, when these are activated, CD31 concentrates at the contact margins of cells in endothelial monolayers. Probably an adhesion molecule.

CD32 (FcγRII; IgG Fc receptor II) See *Fcγ receptors*.

CD35 See *CR1*.

CD36 A membrane glycoprotein found on *mononuclear phagocytes* and *platelets*. *Macrophage* surface CD36 together with a β₃ integrin (the vitronectin

receptor) bind a platelet-derived protein named thrombospondin. This is the basis for a mechanism for ingestion of apoptotic (see *apoptosis*) *neutrophil leucocytes*. These, but not healthy neutrophils, also bind thrombospondin. Thus the neutrophils become cross-linked to, and ingested by, macrophages. CD36 may also bind red cells infected with the malaria parasite *Plasmodium falciparum*.

CD38 A *Type II transmembrane protein*. Found on *germinal centre* B lymphocytes but not on *B lymphocytes* from *primary follicles*, thus is a very useful marker for germinal centres and for cells derived from them. Also found on early forms of *T cells* and B cells. Has activity as ADP-ribosyl cyclase and may mobilize Ca²⁺ through this pathway.

CD39 Found on activated *B lymphocytes* and *NK cells*. It is a useful marker for B cells in *lymphoid tissues* since it is present on follicular mantle (*mantle zone*) and *marginal zone* B cells (see *germinal centre* and *lymph node*) but not on germinal centre cells thus allowing these cell types to be distinguished.

CD40 A *Type I transmembrane protein* of the *TNFR superfamily*. Found on *B lymphocytes* and on *dendritic cells*. In *germinal centres*, T lymphocyte-surface *CD40L* rescues *antigen*-activated B cells from *apoptosis* by binding to CD40. B cells rescued in this way become B memory cells (see *immunological memory*).

CD40L (CD40 ligand) A transmembrane protein that has homology with *TNF-α* and is found on activated but not on resting *T cells*. It derives its name from the fact that it binds to *CD40* on *B cells*, and this binding is essential for induction of proliferation of B cells in response to *antigen* and for the formation of memory (see *immunological memory*) B cells (see also *X-linked hyper-IgM syndrome*).

CD43 (leukosialin; glycophorin) A very heavily glycosylated *Type I transmembrane protein* found on *T lymphocytes* and many other *leucocytes*. Can enhance T cell activation and can bind to

ICAM-1. Expression may be transiently decreased in *Wiskott–Aldrich syndrome*. See Figure C3.

CD44 A *Type I transmembrane protein* found on many cell types and in many tissues. Variants exist due to alternative RNA splicing and post-translational modifications. A low molecular weight variant (MW 80–90 kD) which binds to hyaluronate is found on *T lymphocytes* and *macrophages*. CD44 mediates *lymphocyte* adhesion to vascular endothelium including that of *high endothelial venules*, e.g. in mucosal tissues. This may be indirect by activating other adhesion molecules. CD44 is also an important determinant of invasiveness of tumour cells.

CD45 A large (240 kD) *Type I transmembrane protein* which exists in a number of isoforms of different molecular weights generated by alternative splicing of three *exons* (A, B and C) at the N-terminal end of the extracellular *domain*. The isoform that lacks these exons is called CD45RO. Another important isoform is CD45RA (gene expresses only exon A). *Monocytes* and *neutrophil leucocytes* are mostly CD45RO+. *B lymphocytes* are CD45RA+. In *T lymphocytes, unprimed* (naive) cells are CD45RA+, but following contact with *antigen* they become CD45RO+. The latter cells are large and migrate preferentially into inflammatory sites, so CD45RO is probably an activation marker on T cells. They may later revert back to the CD45RA isoform. The cytoplasmic domain of CD45 has phosphotyrosine phosphatase activity. CD45 binds to *CD22* (a B cell marker). See Figure C3.

CD46 See *membrane cofactor protein*.

CD49 (very late antigens; VLA) A series of proteins (CD49a–f) which are members of the *integrin superfamily* (thus *Type I transmembrane proteins*). They are integrin α chains that form heterodimers with β chains, especially β₁ (*CD29*). Several of these molecules are present on *lymphocytes*, e.g. VLA-4 (CD29/CD49d; α₄β₁) and are usually expressed late after antigen challenge,

hence the name Very Late Antigen. VLA-4 binds to *VCAM-1* on endothelial cells activated by *IL-4* or *IFN*-γ. Other members of the family function chiefly in adhesion to the extracellular matrix.

CD50 (ICAM-3) See *ICAM-1, -2, -3*.

CD54 (ICAM-1) See *ICAM-1, -2, -3*.

CD55 See *decay accelerating factor*.

CD56 A *Type I transmembrane protein* of the *Ig superfamily* found on *NK cells*. CD56 is widely used as a marker for these cells. It is an isoform of N-CAM (neural cell adhesion molecule) found in the central nervous system.

CD58 See *LFA-3*.

CD59 (protectin) A control protein found on the surface of erythrocytes that inhibits insertion of the *membrane attack complex* (q.v.). Lacking in *paroxysmal nocturnal haemoglobinuria* (q.v.).

CD62 See *selectins*. CD62E is E-selectin, CD62L is L-selectin and CD62P is P-selectin.

CD64 (FcγRI) See *Fcγ receptors*.

CD74 See *invariant chain*.

CD77 A glycosphingolipid (globotriaocylceramide) which is found in *germinal centre* B cells undergoing *apoptosis*. It is also a marker for *Burkitt's lymphoma* cells. Binds to various *antigens* from Gram negative bacteria.

CD79 CD79a (Ig-α; MB-1) and CD79b (Ig-β; B29) are two small (22 kD) Type I *Ig superfamily* proteins which are associated with *membrane immunoglobulin* in *B cells*. Together they form a disulphide-linked heterodimer. They are necessary for the expression of membrane *IgM*, and may be associated with other membrane immunoglobulins. They share some sequence homology with *CD3* in *T cells*.

CD80 (B7/BB1) A *Type I transmembrane protein* of the *Ig superfamily*, found on activated *B cells, activated macrophages*

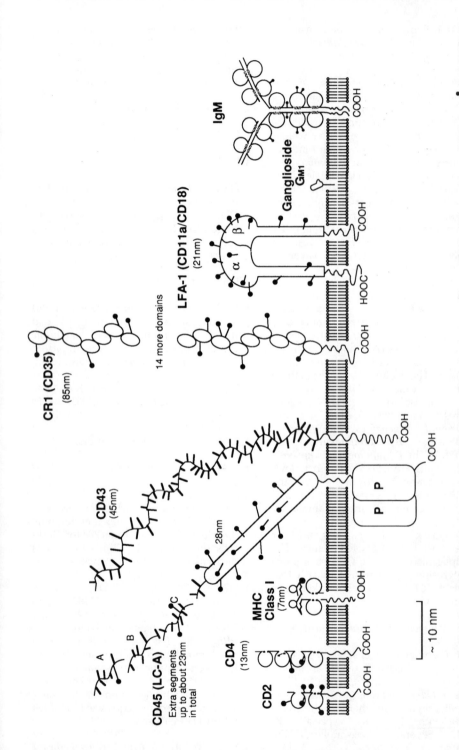

Figure C3. CD antigens. An illustration of the relative size and shape of some common leucocyte surface molecules. The positions of N-linked (†) and O-linked (/) glycosylation sites are indicated but not drawn to scale. 'P' in CD45 indicates the phospho-tyrosine phosphatase cytoplasmic domains. The models are based on data from electron microscopy and X-ray crystallography.

and *dendritic cells*. CD80 is the ligand for *CD28* and for *CTLA-4*, both of which are found on *T cells*. Binding of CD80 to these proteins sends a costimulatory signal to T cells which have already engaged antigen via the T cell receptor (*TCR*).

CD88 (C5aR) See *C5a*.

CD89 See *Fcα receptor*.

CDw90 See *Thy 1*.

CD102 (ICAM-2) See *ICAM-1, -2, -3*.

CD106 See *VCAM-1*.

CD122 (IL-2Rβ) The beta chain of *IL-2R* (q.v.).

CDR (complementarity determining regions) See *hypervariable regions*.

cell cooperation See *T lymphocyte–B lymphocyte cooperation*.

cell-mediated immunity (CMI) *Specific immunity* mediated by *T lymphocytes* which recognize *major histocompatibility complex*-bound *antigens* upon contact with the cells bearing them. This results in proliferation and maturation of the antigen-specific T cells to form T effector cells. Essential in defence against many viral and some bacterial infections. Also important in *allograft* rejection. Activated T cells release *cytokines* with effects on other cell types so that the effector cell of CMI may be a cell other than a T lymphocyte. Cf. *humoral immunity* and *cellular immunity*.

cell-mediated immunity deficiency syndromes Syndromes characterized by failure to express reactions of *cell-mediated immunity*, i.e. to reject a skin *allograft* (see *graft rejection*), become sensitized to agents causing *contact hypersensitivity*, show *delayed-type hypersensitivity* reactions, etc. Examples include *Di George's syndrome, thymic hypoplasia* and *SCID*, q.v.

cellular immunity (1) Term originated by Metchnikoff to refer to an increased ability of phagocytic cells to destroy or to digest parasitic organisms (see *phagocytosis*), and properly so used. Thus is a synonym for macrophage immunity. (2) Sometimes used to refer to *cell-mediated immunity* q.v.

central lymphoid organs Those *lymphoid tissues* (organs) that are essential to the ontogeny of the immune response, i.e. the *thymus* and, in birds, the *bursa of Fabricius*. Cf. *peripheral lymphoid organs*.

centrally acting adjuvants *Adjuvant* substances such as *endotoxin* that stimulate an enhanced *immune response* even when given at a different time or site from the *antigen*. Cf. *depot forming adjuvants*.

centroblast A large *B lymphocyte* found chiefly in the dark zone of *germinal centres* during *immune responses*. The *immunoglobulin genes* of centroblasts undergo *somatic hypermutation*. The cells are also in process of *isotype switching* and have lost *membrane immunoglobulin*. They develop into smaller *centrocytes* which migrate into the light zone of the germinal centre.

centrocyte A non-dividing *B cell* found in *germinal centres*. They derive from *centroblasts* and have a characteristic cleft nucleus. Centrocytes have undergone *isotype switching*, and re-express *membrane immunoglobulin*, i.e. mIgG and mIgA. They migrate across the light zone of the germinal centre to make contact with antigen-bearing *follicular dendritic cells*. Those with high *affinity* for the *antigen* are positively selected (see *positive selection*) and go on to become *antibody*-secreting *plasma cells* or B memory cells (see *immunological memory*) depending on the costimulatory signals that they receive (see *CD40, CD40L*). The unselected cells die and are removed by *tingible body macrophages*.

Table C1. CD antigens. (A list of abbreviations and notes will be found at the end of this table)

Molecule	Superfamily or other structural features	Other names	Major cell distribution	Comment
CD1a, 1b, 1c	Ig		Cortical Thy, DC	*See entry*
CD2	Ig	LFA-2	T, NK	*See entry*
CD3	Ig	TCR/CD3	T	*See entry*
CD4	Ig		T$_H$, Mono, MΦ	*See entry*
CD5	Scavenger R		T, B-1 subset	*See entry*
CD6	Scavenger R		T, Thy	
CD7	Ig		T, Thy	
CD8	Ig		CTL	*See entry*
CD9	TM4		Plat, pre-B, T, Eos, Bas	
CD10		CALLA	PMN, Immature T & B	*See entry*
CD11a	Integrin	α$_L$ (LFA-1)	Most leucocytes	*See entry*
CD11b	Integrin	α$_M$ (MAC-1, CR3)	PMN, Mono, MΦ, NK	*See entry*
CD11c	Integrin	α$_x$ (p150:95)	PMN, Mono, MΦ, DC	*See entry*
CDw12			PMN, Mono, Plat	
CD13			PMN, Eos, Bas, Mono	Aminopeptidase N
CD14	GPI anchor		Mono, MΦ, PMN	*See entry*
CD15		Lewis x	PMN	*See entry*
CD15s		Sialyl Lewis x	PMN, Mono	See CD15 entry
CD16a	Ig	FcγRIII	MΦ, NK	See *Fcγ receptor*
CD16b	Ig (GPI anchor)	FcγRIII	PMN	See *Fcγ receptor*
CDw17			PMN, Mono, Plat	Lactosylceramide
CD18	Integrin	β$_2$ chain	Most leucocytes	*See entry*
CD19	Ig		B, B precursors	*See entry*
CD20			B, pre-B	*See entry*
CD21	SCR	CR2	B, FDC	See *CR2*
CD22	Ig		B, B precursors	*See entry*
CD23	C-type lectin	FcεRII	Mature, B, FDC, MΦ, Eos, Mono	*See entry*
CD24	GPI anchor		B, B precursors	B cell maturation
CD25	SCR	Tac, IL-2Rα	Activated, T, B	See *IL-2R*
CD26			Many cells inc. T	Cofactor for entry of *HIV*. Dipeptidyl peptidase
CD27	TNFR		T, Thy	Costimulatory, binds CD70
CD28	Ig		Activated T	*See entry*
CD29	Integrin	β$_1$ chain	Most cells	*See entry*
CD30	TNFR		Activated T, B, Reed–Sternberg cells	See *Hodgkin's disease*
CD31	Ig	PECAM	Endo, Plat, Mono, MΦ, PMN	*See entry*
CD32	Ig	FcγRII	Mono, MΦ, PMN, Eos, B	See *Fcγ receptor*
CD33	Ig		Mono, Myeloid precursors	

Continued

Table C1. Continued

Molecule	Superfamily or other structural features	Other names	Major cell distribution	Comment
CD34			Endo, Haemopoietic precursors	Heavily glycosylated
CD35	SCR	CR1	B, Mono, MΦ, PMN, Eos, FDC	*See* **CR1**
CD36		Platelet glycoprotein IV	Plat, Mono	*See entry*
CD37	TM4		Mature B	
CD38			Immature T B, Germinal centre B	*See entry*
CD39			Mature B, NK, some T, DC	*See entry*
CD40	TNFR		Mature B, DC	*See entry*
CD41	Integrin	α_{IIb} chain	Plat	Platelet adhesion, aggregation
CD42			Plat	Platelet adhesion
CD43		Leukosialin, sialophorin	Most leucocytes	*See entry*
CD44			Many leucocytes	*See entry*
CD45		LCA	All leucocytes	*See entry*
CD46	SCR	MCP	Most leucocytes	*See* **membrane cofactor protein**
CD47			Most leucocytes	Associates with **integrins**
CD48	Ig (GPI anchor)	MRC OX-45	Most leucocytes	Sequence similarity to CD2, CD58. Possibly costimulatory
CD49(a–f)	Integrin	α chains of VLA 1–6	Many leucocytes	*See entry*
CD50	Ig	ICAM-3	Most leucocytes	*See* **ICAM**
CD51	Integrin	α_v-chain, vitronectin-receptor	Plat, Endo	Adhesion to extracellular matrix
CDw52	GPI anchor	CAMPATH-1	T, Thy, B, Eos	Target for **complement**-mediated lysis
CD53	TM4	MRC OX-44	Most leucocytes	Possible transport molecule
CD54	Ig	ICAM-1	Endo, Activated T, B, Mono	*See entry*
CD55	SCR (GPI anchor)	DAF	Wide distribution	*See* **decay accelerating factor**
CD56	Ig		NK, some T	*See entry*
CD57	Oligosaccharide		NK, some T & B	Oligosaccharide epitope associated with various proteins
CD58	Ig	LFA-3	Most leucocytes	*See* **LFA-3**
CD59	GPI anchor	Protectin	Wide distribution	*See entry*

Continued

Table C1. Continued

Molecule	Superfamily or other structural features	Other names	Major cell distribution	Comment
CDw60	Oligosaccharide epitope		Mono, Plat, some T	
CD61	Integrin	GPIIIa, β_3 chain	Plat, MΦ	Platelet adhesion
CD62E	SCR	E selectin	Wide cell distribution	See *selectins*
CD62L	SCR	L selectin	Wide cell distribution	See *selectins*
CD62P	SCR	P selectin	Wide cell distribution	See *selectins*
CD63	TM4		Activated Plat, Mono, PMN	Platelet activation. Neutrophil and monocyte adhesion
CD64	Ig	FcγRI	Mono, MΦ, Activated PMN	See *Fcγ receptor*
CDw65	Glycolipid		PMN, Mono	
CD66 (a to e)	Ig (GPI anchor)	Carcino-embryonic antigen (CD66e)	PMN, colonic epithelium	Probably adhesion
CD67	No protein presently assigned to this number. Previous CD67 is now CD66b			
CD68	Lysosomal glycoprotein	Macrosialin	Mono, MΦ, Plat, PMN, Bas	
CD69			Activated T, activated B, MΦ, activated NK	Activation antigen in lymphocytes
CD70	TNF		Activated T, activated B, Reed–Sternberg cells	Ligand for CD27. Costimulatory for T cells
CD71		Transferrin receptor	Proliferating cells of all types	
CD72	C-type lectin		B, B precursors	Binds CD5. Has sequence homology with CD23
CD73	GPI anchor		B, some T, Endo	Ecto-5'-nucleotidase. Activity is low in various immunodeficiencies
CD74		Invariant chain	Class II MHC antigen-positive cells	See *invariant chain*
CDw75			Mature B, some T	May bind CD22
CDw76	Carbohydrate epitope		B (*mantle zone*), some T	
CD77	Glycosphingolipid	Globotriaocyl-ceramide	Germinal centre B, Burkitt's lymphoma cells	See *entry*
CDw78			B	
CD79(a & b)	Ig	Ig-α and Ig-β	B	See *entry*
CD80	Ig	B7/BB1	Activated B, DC, MΦ	See *entry*

Continued

Table C1. Continued

Molecule	Superfamily or other structural features	Other names	Major cell distribution	Comment
CD81	TM4	TAPA-1	B, T, NK, Eos	
CD82	TM4		Many cells	
CD83			DC, Langerhans' cells	Specific marker for *dendritic cells*
CDw84			Mono, MΦ, Plat	
CD85			Plasma cells, Mono	
CD86		FUN-1	Germinal centre B, Mono	
CD87			Myeloid cells	Urokinase plasminogen activator receptor
CD88	Rhodopsin	C5aR	PMN, Mono, MΦ	See *C5a*
CD89	Ig	FcαR	PMN, Mono, MΦ, some B, T	See *Fca receptor*
CDw90	Ig (GPI anchor)	Thy-1	T, Thy, brain	See *Thy-1*
CD91			Mono, MΦ	α_2-macroglobulin receptor
CDw92			PMN, Mono, Endo, Plat	
CD93			PMN, Mono, Endo	
CD94			NK, αβ and γδ T subsets	
CD95	TNFR	APO-1, Fas	Many cell types	See *Fas*
CD96		TACTILE	Activated T, and activated NK	T cell ACTivated. Increased Late Expression
CD97	TNFR		Activated cells	
CD98			Wide distribution	
CD99		MIC2	Thy, T, B	Can form rosettes with *SRBC*
CD100			Many	
CDw101			CD28+ T, PMN, Mono	
CD102	Ig	ICAM-2	T, B, Mono, Plat, Endo	See *ICAM*
CD103	Integrin	HML-1, α_E integrin chain	*Intraepithelial lymphocytes* and other mucosal cells	Human mucosal lymphocyte integrin (α_E/β_7), *MAdCAM* receptor
CD104	Integrin	β_4 chain	Thy, epithelial cells	
CD105			Endo, Activated Mono	Receptor for *TGF-β*
CD106	Ig	VCAM-1	Endo	See *VCAM-1*
CD107(a & b)		LAMP-1 & 2	Activated Plat	Lysosomal associated membrane protein
CDw108	GPI anchor		Activated T	
CDw109	GPI anchor		Activated T, Activated Plat, Endo	

Continued

Table C1. Continued

Molecule	Superfamily or other structural features	Other names	Major cell distribution	Comment
CD110		No protein presently assigned to this number		
CD111		No protein presently assigned to this number		
CD112		No protein presently assigned to this number		
CD113		No protein presently assigned to this number		
CD114		No protein presently assigned to this number		
CD115	Ig	M-CSFR	Mono, MΦ, myeloid precursors	See *M-CSFR*
CDw116	Cytokine R	GM-CSFR	Mono, PMN, Eos, myeloid precursors	See *GM-CSF*
CD117	Ig	c-Kit, SCFR	Bone marrow progenitors	See *C-Kit*
CD118		Reserved for IFN-α/IFN-β receptor		
CDw119		IFN-γR	Mono, MΦ, B	See *IFN-γ*
CD120(a & b)	TNFR	TNFR I and II	Wide specificity	See *TNFR-I & II*
CDw121	Ig	IL-1R	T, B, MΦ, Mono	See *IL-1R*
CD122	Cytokine R	IL-2Rβ	T, NK, Mono	See *IL-2R*
CD123		Reserved for *IL-3R*		
CDw124	Cytokine R	IL-4R	T, B	See *IL-4R*
CD125		Reserved for *IL-5R*		
CD126	Cytokine R and Ig	IL-6R	Activated B	See *IL-6R*
CDw127		IL-7R	Pro B, Thy, T	See *IL-7*
CDw128	Rhodopsin	IL-8R	PMN, some T, Bas	See *chemokine receptors*
CD129		Reserved for IL-9R		
CDw130		gp-130 IL-6R-associated IL-11R-associated	Many cells	Associates with CD126

CD molecules which have been defined in the text of the Dictionary are indicated in *bold/italic* and the reader is referred to those definitions for more detail. Other molecules, e.g. CD21, may be defined under a different name, e.g. *CR2* and these are indicated similarly.
Abbreviations: B, *B cell*; Bas, *basophil leucocyte*; CTL, *cytotoxic T lymphocyte*; DC, *dendritic cell*; Endo, vascular endothelium; Eos, *eosinophil leuocyte*; FDC, *follicular dendritic cell*; Mono, *monocyte*; MΦ, *macrophage*; NK, *NK cell*; Plat, *platelet*; PMN, *neutrophil leucocyte*; T, *T cell*; Thy, *thymocyte*; TM4, Transmembrane 4 pass superfamily (*TM4 superfamily*).

CFA See *complete Freund's adjuvant*.

CFT See *complement fixation test*.

CFU See *colony forming unit*.

CGD See *chronic granulomatous disease*.

C$_H$ The *constant region* of the *heavy chain* of *immunoglobulin*.

C$_H$1, C$_H$2, C$_H$3, C$_H$4 Designations given to the *homology regions* (*immunoglobulin domains* q.v.) of the *constant region* of the *heavy chain* of *immunoglo-*bulins. Each heavy chain is made up of a number of homology regions named (starting at the N-terminal end) C$_H$1, C$_H$2, etc. In *IgG* C$_H$1 forms the constant half of the *Fab fragment* and C$_H$2 and C$_H$3 form the *Fc fragment*. *IgM* has a longer heavy chain with an extra homology region C$_H$4. Commonly given the corresponding Greek letter of the heavy chain, e.g. C$_\mu$1, C$_\mu$2, etc.

CH$_{50}$ In immune haemolysis, the dose of *complement* which is capable of lysing 50% of a test suspension of red cells coated with anti red cell antibody.

challenge (1) Administration of *antigen* to provoke an *immunological reaction*[1]. Usually used of the second or later doses of antigen. (2) Administration of a virulent pathogen, e.g. in order to test initial *immunity* or the degree of protection achieved by *vaccination*.

chaperonins See *heat shock proteins*.

Chediak–Higashi syndrome Disease of children inherited as autosomal recessive. The children show an increased susceptibility to severe pyogenic infection. There is a defect of granulopoiesis and the *neutrophil leucocytes* contain abnormally large *lysosomal* granules or *phagolysosomes* and are defective in microbicidal and chemotactic function. There is also a defect of *NK cell* function. In some cases the syndrome is characterized by pale skin, hair and eyes due to lack of formation of melanin. Similar syndromes are seen in a number of species, e.g. the *beige mouse*.

chemiluminescence Emission of photons as a result of chemical reactions. In immunological contexts, measurement of chemiluminescence is a useful measure of the oxidative generation of free radicals (see *reactive oxygen intermediates*) by *neutrophil leucocytes* and *mononuclear phagocytes* (and possibly *NK cells*). A rapid burst of chemiluminescence can be detected following the addition to these cells of phagocytosable particles (see *phagocytosis*), chemotactic factors (see *chemotaxis*) or other excitatory entities.

chemoattractant Any molecule that stimulates *leucocyte* locomotion, whether by *chemotaxis* or *chemokinesis* or both.

chemokine receptors *Type III transmembrane proteins* of the *rhodopsin superfamily* (seven membrane-spanning domains). (a) Receptors for α-*chemokines*. Two receptors, IL-8RA (*CDw128*) and IL-8RB, have been identified on *neutrophil leucocytes*. IL-8RA is selective for *IL-8*. IL-8RB binds IL-8 and other α-chemokines, e.g. NAP-2, GRO. (b) Receptors for β-chemokines. There

are at least three β-chemokine receptors which overlap in *ligand* binding; (i) a receptor that binds *MCP-1* and *MCP-3*; (ii) a receptor that binds RANTES and MCP-3; and (iii) a receptor that binds *MIP-1α* and RANTES. (c) A broad specificity receptor for both classes of chemokine is found on erythrocytes. This spans the membrane nine times (thus unrelated to rhodopsin), carries the Duffy *blood group* antigen, and is the *binding site* for the malarial parasite *Plasmodium vivax*.

chemokines A family of *cytokines* with cell-specific chemoattractant activity (see *chemotaxis*) and other activating properties for various cell types within the immune system. See Table C2. There are two subfamilies, the α-chemokines and the β-chemokines. As monomers they are 8 kD proteins, but different members may normally be found as dimers or multimers.

(a) **The α-chemokines**, of which the first described was *IL-8*, are sometimes known as the C-X-C chemokines because of a characteristic sequence of two cysteines separated by a single variable intervening residue. They are activators of *neutrophil leucocyte* functions including chemotaxis, have no activity for *mononuclear phagocytes*, but some may have less well-studied effects on other immune cells, e.g. *lymphocytes*.

(b) **The β-chemokines** are also known as the C-C chemokines because the above-mentioned cysteine residues are adjacent. These have chemoattractant and other activating effects on *monocytes* and *macrophages*, but not on neutrophil leucocytes. Various members of the subfamily also stimulate *T lymphocytes*, *eosinophil leucocytes* and *basophil leucocytes*.

Note that cytokines other than the chemokine family may also be chemotactic factors for a variety of cell types, e.g. *TGF-β* and *TNF* for mononuclear phagocytes, *IL-5* for eosinophils, *IL-2* and *IL-15* for T lymphocytes.

chemokinesis A reaction by which the speed of locomotion and/or the frequency of random turning of cells or organisms is determined by substances in their environment. Chemokinesis

Table C2. Cell-specific chemoattractant activities of chemokines

	Neutrophil	Monocyte/ macrophage	T lymphocyte (activated)	Basophil	Eosinophil
α-chemokines					
IL-8	+	−	+	∓	
NAP-2	+	−	−		
GRO	+	−			
ENA-78	+	−			
β-TG	−	−			
(inactive precursor of NAP-2)					
PF-4	−	−			
MIP-2	+	−			
β-chemokines					
MCP-1	−	+	−	+	−
MCP-2	−	+			
MCP-3	−	+		+	+
MIP-1α	−	+	±	∓	∓
MIP-1β	−	+	∓	−	∓
RANTES	−	+	∓	+	+

IL-8, interleukin 8; MCP, monocyte chemotactic protein; MIP, macrophage inflammatory protein; NAP, neutrophil activating protein; PF-4, platelet factor 4; RANTES, Regulation upon Activation Normal T cell Expressed and Secreted; β-TG, β-thromboglobulin; ENA-78 and GRO are only named as acronyms.

does not determine the direction of migration of cells (cf. *chemotaxis*). Leucocytes show chemokinesis when exposed to uniform concentrations of the chemical substances listed under chemotaxis, but physical constraints, e.g. adhesion, as well as chemical signals also determine the speed at which cells move.

chemotaxis Reaction by which the direction of locomotion and the orientation of cells is determined by chemical substances. The cells become oriented and move towards (positive chemotaxis) or away from (negative chemotaxis) the source of a concentration gradient of the substance. Leucocytes (*neutrophil* and *eosinophil leucocytes, monocytes* and *lymphocytes*) show positive chemotaxis towards many agents including *C5a, formyl peptides, leukotriene* B₄, *chemokines* and other *cytokines*, bacterial substances and products of cell damage or denatured proteins. Essential for recruitment of cells to sites of tissue injury and inflammation.

chimera (chimaera) A fire-breathing monster of Greek mythology – with lion's head, goat's body and serpent's tail. Immunology: An animal containing a mixture of cells derived from two individuals of different genotype. Such animals occur naturally (rarely) due to the fusion of the placental blood circulatory systems of dizygotic twins *in utero*. They have been observed in humans and cows, see *freemartin*. Chimeras can also be produced artificially, see *tetraparental chimera* and *irradiation chimera*. The term is also used to describe a form of *humanized antibody* where the *variable regions* of rodent *antibodies* are grafted onto the *constant regions* of human antibodies.

chimerism A state in which two or more genetically different populations of cells coexist. See *chimera* and *irradiation chimera*.

chromium release assay *In vitro* test in which cells are labelled with a radioisotope of chromium (⁵¹Cr) and used as targets for antibody-dependent or cell-mediated cytotoxicity (see *antibody-dependent cell-mediated cytotoxicity* and *cytotoxic T lymphocyte*). Radiolabel is released in proportion to the number of cells killed.

chronic granulocytic leukaemia The commonest form of *chronic myeloid leukaemia* in which the Philadelphia chromosome abnormality is present.

chronic granulomatous disease (CGD) Disease due to a defect in oxidative microbicidal activity in *neutrophil leucocytes* and characterized by recurrent suppurative inflammation of *lymph nodes*, pulmonary *granulomata* and visceral abscesses with anaemia, *leucocytosis* and raised serum *immunoglobulin* levels. There is a defect in the genes that regulate the NADPH oxidase which mediates electron transport necessary for the generation of microbicidal *reactive oxygen intermediates*. Thus, while the neutrophils are able to ingest bacteria, they are unable to kill them. The commonest form is X-linked, occurs in boys and the defect is in the gene for cytochrome b. Other non X-linked variants involve defects in genes for control proteins for cytochrome b.

chronic lymphocytic leukaemia (CLL) Leukaemia, commonest in the elderly, characterized by large numbers of *lymphocytes* in the blood and *lymphoid tissues*. In the majority of cases, these are monoclonal, non-reactive, *B lymphocytes* (*CD5+, CD23+ B-1 lymphocytes*) which carry *membrane immunoglobulins IgM* and *IgD*. The *T lymphocyte* form is rare.

chronic mucocutaneous candidiasis A systemic disease characterized by a persistent *Candida albicans* infection affecting mainly the skin, nails and mucosae. Associated with endocrine abnormalities and immunological defects, e.g. defective *cell-mediated immune* responses to *Candida antigens*.

chronic myeloid leukaemia A leukaemia characterized by the presence of high numbers of *neutrophil leucocytes* and their precursors (especially myelocytes) in the blood. Probably arises from clonal expansion of an abnormal *stem cell*, thus leukaemic cells of lineages other than the *myeloid cell*

series (e.g. *lymphoblasts*) may appear, particularly late in the disease. Most patients have a chromosomal abnormality (the Philadelphia chromosome) with a translocation of part of chromosomes 9 and 22 (chronic granulocytic leukaemia). Forms of chronic myeloid leukaemia are also seen in which blood *monocyte* levels are raised (chronic myelomonocytic leukaemia).

cisternal space The lumen of the *endoplasmic reticulum* (ER) or of the Golgi apparatus. In *plasma cells* the ER cisternal space contains *immunoglobulin* molecules and subunits destined for secretion.

C_L The *constant region* of the *light chain* of *immunoglobulin*. Commonly given the Greek letter corresponding to the light chain *isotype*, i.e. C_κ, C_λ.

class I MHC antigens Histocompatibility antigens composed of two noncovalently associated *Type I transmembrane proteins*; a heavy chain of MW 44 kD linked to β_2 *microglobulin*, MW 12 kD (structure shown in Figure C4). β_2 microglobulin is identical in all class I antigens and is the product of a separate chromosome from that coding for the heavy chain, which is the product of the *major histocompatibility complex*. The heavy chain exhibits extensive polymorphism and is coded for by the K, D and L genes of the mouse H-2 complex and the A, B and C genes of the human HLA complex (see maps of the H-2 and HLA genes, Figures H1 and H2). Class I antigens are expressed on the surface membranes of all nucleated cells (see Figure C3) and their function is to present antigenic peptides to class I *MHC restricted, T cells*. The heavy chain consists of three extracellular domains (α_1, α_2 and α_3) of which the outer two (α_1 and α_2) form an antigen-binding groove. This cleft in the surface of the protein has side walls consisting of α helical loops and a platformlike floor composed of β-pleated sheets. The groove accommodates peptides of 8–9 amino acids in length.

class II MHC antigens Histocompatibility antigens composed of two noncovalently associated *Type I transmem-*

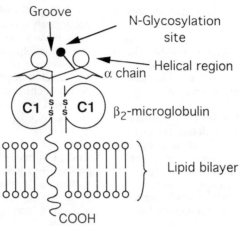

Figure C4. Class I antigen.

brane proteins: α chain, MW 32 kD and β chain, MW 28 kD. (Structure shown in Figure C5). Class II MHC antigens are expressed predominantly on *dendritic cells, B lymphocytes, macrophages* and other *accessory cells*, but are inducible on other cells including epithelium and vascular endothelium. Their function is to present antigenic peptides to class II *MHC restricted T cells*, with the outer α_1 and β_1 *domains* forming an antigen-binding groove similar to, but larger than, that in class I MHC molecules. The murine class II MHC region includes loci Aα, Aβ, $E\beta_2$ and Eα coding for the

relevant α and β chains (see H-2 gene map Figure H1), while the human class II MHC locus contains the genes coding the α and β chains of the HLA-DR, HLA-DP and HLA-DQ molecules (see **HLA histocompatibility system** and Figure H2).

class switching See *isotype switching*.

classical complement pathway The pathway of *complement* activation that commences with the binding of C1q (see *C1*) to an *antibody–antigen* complex followed by the activation of C1, *C4* and

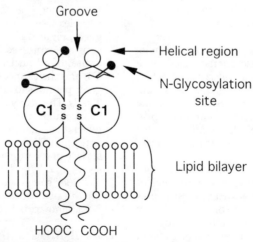

Figure C5. Class II antigen.

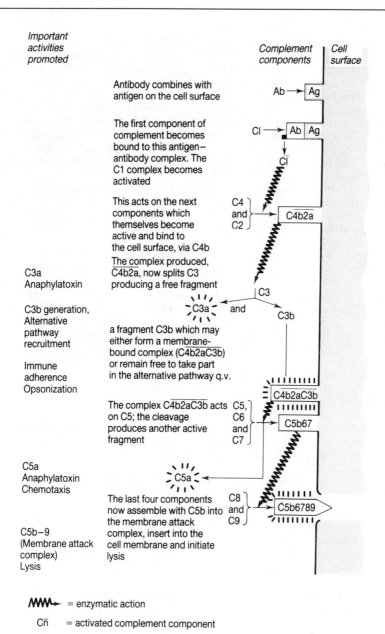

Figure C6. Classical complement pathway.

The figure is labelled with the following text:

Important activities promoted

Complement components | Cell surface

Antibody combines with antigen on the cell surface — Ab → Ag

The first component of complement becomes bound to this antigen–antibody complex. The C1 complex becomes activated — Cl → Ab | Ag → C̄l

This acts on the next components which themselves become active and bind to the cell surface, via C4b — C4 and C2 → C4b2a

C3a Anaphylatoxin

The complex produced, C4b2a, now splits C3 producing a free fragment — C3 → C3a and C3b

C3b generation, Alternative pathway recruitment

a fragment C3b which may either form a membrane-bound complex (C4b2aC3b) or remain free to take part in the alternative pathway q.v.

Immune adherence Opsonization — C4b2aC3b

The complex C4b2aC3b acts on C5; the cleavage produces another active fragment — C5, C6 and C7 → C5b67

C5a Anaphylatoxin Chemotaxis — C5a

The last four components now assemble with C5b into the membrane attack complex, insert into the cell membrane and initiate lysis — C8 and C9 → C5b6789

C5b–9 (Membrane attack complex) Lysis

〜〜→ = enzymatic action

C̄n = activated complement component

C2, see Figure C6. Cf. *alternative pathway*.

clonal anergy See *anergy*.

clonal deletion *Programmed cell death* of inappropriately stimulated clones of antigen-reactive *lymphocytes*. See *immunological tolerance*, *negative selection*.

clonal selection theory A *selective theory of the immune response* proposed by Burnet. According to this theory, the normal individual carries a complement of clones of *lymphocytes* capable of reacting with all possible *epitopes*. During fetal life, those clones reactive against *autoantigens* are eliminated or rendered anergic (see *anergy*) on contact with *antigen* resulting in *immunological tolerance*. After birth, a change in the response to contact with antigen occurs, so that the normal response is proliferation, *antibody* production and *cell-mediated immunity*. Some self-reactive clones persist in an anergic state and become active in later life leading to *autoimmune disease*. This theory is now generally accepted as an accurate description of the immune system in broad outline.

clonotype The pattern of bands, produced by *isoelectric focusing* (q.v.), of *immunoglobulin* secreted by a clone of *B cells*. Although the primary amino acid sequence of each immunoglobulin molecule is identical, microheterogeneity is caused mainly by variation in the number of sialic acid residues, resulting in several bands in a pattern, or 'fingerprint', unique to that clone. Used to determine the number and behaviour of B cell clones during an *immune response*. See also *reverse immunoblotting*.

CMI See *cell-mediated immunity*.

cNOS (constitutive nitric oxide synthase) See *nitric oxide*.

co-precipitation See *coprecipitation*.

co-stimulatory molecules See *costimulatory molecules*.

co-operation See *T lymphocyte–B lymphocyte cooperation*.

cobra venom The venom of the Indian cobra, *Naja naja*. It contains a factor ('cobra venom factor') which is the cobra analogue of *C3b*. It therefore activates the *alternative pathway* to *complement activation* in the same way as does human C3b. Cobra venoms also contain many other biologically active factors including phospholipase A.

coeliac disease A malabsorption syndrome with characteristic histology of the proximal small intestine, i.e. subtotal villous atrophy, lymphocytic infiltration of the epithelium and crypt hyperplasia. Patients have serum and intestinal *antibodies* to gluten, and the malabsorption and the morphological lesions improve when glutens are excluded from the diet. The condition is strongly associated with the presence of certain *class II MHC antigens* (HLA-DQ2) and appears to be due to a *T lymphocyte*-mediated *immune response* to gluten derived from wheat or rye.

coelomocyte Generic term used in invertebrate biology for circulating and sessile *leucocytes* involved in internal defence mechanisms such as *phagocytosis* and encapsulation, in animals such as earthworms and echinoderms whose body-cavity is embryologically derived from the mesoderm (coelom). See also *haemocyte*.

coisogenic strain See *congenic strain* (synonym).

cold antibody Any *antibody* serologically (see *serology*) detectable at a higher *titre* below 37°C than at 37°C.

cold haemoglobinuria See *paroxysmal cold haemoglobinuria*.

collagen induced arthritis Experimental model of *autoimmune* arthritis induced by injection of type II collagen, the predominant form in articular cartilage.

collectins A family of carbohydrate-binding oligomeric proteins with collagen-like structures and C-terminal *lectin* domains hence the name from col(lagen) and lectin. Includes pulmonary surfactant proteins, *conglutinin*, and *mannose-binding protein* (q.v.). The lectin *domain* binds to microbial carbohydrates while the collagen domains bind to receptors on *phagocytes* thus acting as *opsonins* and also activating *complement*.

colony forming unit In cultures of haemopoietic tissues (*bone marrow,* *spleen*, etc.), a single cell which gives rise to a colony of daughter cells is called a colony forming cell or colony forming unit. Such cells may give rise to discrete populations, e.g. of cells from the *myeloid cell series*, or to mixed populations, depending on the maturation status of the precursor cell.

colony stimulating factors (CSF) *Cytokines* that control the growth and maturation of the precursors of the cells of the immune system, including *stem cells* and the precursors of the *myeloid cell series* and *lymphoid cell series* as well as other cells of the blood. Different colony stimulating factors act at different levels, for example *GM-CSF* commits precursors to the myeloid cell line and *G-CSF* and *M-CSF* later determine whether they will become *granulocytes* or *monocytes*. Colony stimulating factors also have many effects on the functions of mature *leucocytes*. See *IL-3*, *IL-5*.

colostrum The first milk produced by the mother post partum. Viscid and yellow with high protein and high *immunoglobulin* content. Source of passive *maternal immunity* in newborn of many species (not man).

combined immunodeficiency See *SCID*.

combining site See *antigen-binding site*.

committed cell Cell committed to a particular differentiation pathway or line of development. In the *bone marrow*, committed cells arise from multipotential *stem cells* and themselves form precursor lines for the various blood cells.

common variable antibody deficiency See *common variable immunodeficiency*.

common variable immunodeficiency A heterogeneous group of *immunodeficiencies* which may present at any age. Ill-defined, but patients often have low *serum* levels of *IgG* and *IgA* but normal levels of *IgM*. Defects of *cell-mediated*

immunity may also be detectable, and the patients may suffer from a wide variety of infections.

complement A system of at least 18 serum proteins and a group of membrane proteins which interact in a complex *cascade reaction* sequence. This leads to the production of important biological effects and substances. These include *haemolysis*, *phagocytosis*, *opsonization*, prevention of *immune complex* formation, immune complex removal, *chemotaxis* and production of *anaphylatoxins* and formation of the *membrane attack complex*. The components of the system are designated as numbers, e.g. *C1* or as names, i.e. *Factor B*. The *classical complement pathway* (Figure C6) is activated primarily by immune complexes formed when *antibody* combines with *antigen*. The *alternative pathway* (Figure A1) is activated by bacterial *endotoxin*, fungal and plant factors. Antigen-specific antibody is not required for initiation of this pathway. Both pathways allow the formation of the *membrane attack complex*, the insertion of which into cell membranes causes severe perturbation or holes resulting in an inability of the cell to survive. It should be noted that some species, notably pig, horse, dog and mouse, have complements that are not as haemolytically active as guinea pig or human complement.

complement activation (complement fixation) The activation of the *complement* system, characteristically by the interaction of *antigen* and *antibody*. The classical sequence of complement fixation is that followed in *immune haemolysis* in which the complement factors *C1–C9* are activated sequentially in a *cascade reaction*, the end result being lysis of the erythrocyte at whose surface, antigen, antibody and complement have interacted. See also *alternative pathway*.

complement control protein superfamily (CCP superfamily) See *SCR superfamily*.

complement deficiency states Hereditary deficiencies of individual components of *complement*. Patients with deficiencies of most of the complement components have now been described. The genes responsible for some of the complement components are located in the human *major histocompatibility complex* between D(R) and B on the 6th chromosome (see Figure H2). Deficiencies of *classical complement pathway* components are associated with *immune complex diseases*, whilst those of the *alternative pathway* and *membrane attack complex* with meningococcal disease. *C3* deficiency gives rise to a severe immunodeficiency with an increased tendency to infection. *C1 inhibitor* deficiency is associated with *hereditary angio-oedema*. Complement deficiencies also occur in laboratory animals, e.g. *C6* deficient rabbits, and especially in inbred strains of mice, e.g. *C5* deficient mice.

complement fixation An older synonym for *complement activation*.

complement fixation inhibition test An *inhibition test*[2] in which the presence of a substance of known structure inhibits the reaction of *antibody* with a complex *antigen* and thus the fixation of complement (see *complement activation*). See also *hapten inhibition test*.

complement fixation test Serological test for the detection of *antibody* which, on reacting with *antigen*, binds (fixes, or activates) *complement*. A two-stage test in which, firstly, antigen, complement (usually guinea pig serum complement) and the *heat inactivated* serum under test are incubated together. Secondly, when this reaction has taken place, an indicator system consisting of sheep red cells coated with anti sheep red cell antibody. In the presence of remaining free complement these cells will lyse. Failure of the cells to lyse indicates that the complement has been fixed in the first reaction and indicates a positive result. The test can also be used (especially in virology) to detect and identify an antigen by using a known *antiserum*.

complement fixing antibody *Antibody* (usually of *immunoglobulin*

classes IgG and *IgM*) which, in reacting with *antigen*, binds (activates) *complement*. Detectable by *complement fixation test*.

complement inhibitors Four naturally occurring serum protein inhibitors of *complement* components are known. These are *C1 inhibitor, Factor I, Factor H* and *C4 binding protein* (C4BP). In addition many substances are used *in vitro* to inhibit complement or its fractions, e.g. hydrazine and ammonia which inhibit *C3* and *C4*, and *heat inactivation* which destroys *C1* and *C2*. Also a purified *cobra venom* fraction or *zymosan* activate *C3* via the *alternative pathway* and thus deplete the plasma of C3.

complementarity determining regions The *hypervariable regions* of *immunoglobulin* molecules. The amino acid sequences in these regions determine the specificity of *antigen* binding.

complete Freund's adjuvant A water-in-oil emulsion *adjuvant* in which killed, dried, mycobacteria (usually *M. tuberculosis*) are suspended in the oil phase. Especially effective in stimulating *cell-mediated immunity*, and in some animals, e.g. guinea pig, potentiates production of certain *immunoglobulin classes*. Cf. *incomplete Freund's adjuvant*.

Con A See *concanavalin A*.

concanavalin A (Con A) A *lectin* derived from the jack bean *Canavalia ensiformis* which binds to glucopyranosides, mannopyranosides and fructofuranosides. Since these are common constituents of cell membrane glycoproteins, Con A binds to membranes containing such glycoproteins. Con A is a tetramer with four binding sites for saccharide and, therefore, acts as a polyvalent ligand to form clusters of protein on the cell membrane. It *agglutinates* cells of many types and acts as a *mitogen*, especially of *T lymphocytes*.

concomitant immunity Resistance to reinfection by a parasite or the fresh establishment of a tumour by a host already infected with the parasite or bearing the tumour. The primary growth, however, is apparently unaffected by the *immune response* which destroys the *challenge* organisms or tumour cells. The term was originally used in tumour immunology but is now used widely in *immunity* to parasites, especially in schistosomiasis.

congenic strain (coisogenic strain) One of a number of separate strains of animals (e.g. mice) all constructed to possess identical genotypes except for a difference at a single gene locus. Although these strains are constructed to be genetically identical outside the single defined locus, the phenomena of mutation and genetic linkage ensure that mice within and between congenic strains will differ randomly at a minority of other foci.

conglutination Agglutination of *antibody*-coated cells in the presence of (non-haemolytic) *complement* and *conglutinin*.

conglutinin Protein of the *collectins* protein family (q.v.) present in serum of Bovidae which can bind to *complement* (*C3b*)-bearing *immune complexes* in the presence of divalent cations. Not an *antibody* and not to be confused with *immunoconglutinin* q.v.

conjugate The product obtained by joining two or more dissimilar molecules by covalent bonds. In immunological contexts, one is usually a protein and the other either a *hapten* or else a label such as *fluorescein*, *ferritin*, or an enzyme (see *ELISA*).

constant region The C-terminal portion of the *heavy chain* containing *homology regions* (*immunoglobulin domains*) C_H1, C_H2, C_H3, etc., or the C-terminal half of the *light chain* of an *immunoglobulin* molecule. So-called because the amino acid sequence in this region is constant from molecule to molecule except for amino acids at *allotype* marker sites. Many other members of the *Ig superfamily* contain domains homologous to the constant regions of immunoglobulin.

contact dermatitis Any inflammatory change in the skin due to exposure, usually repeated, to chemical substances. One form, *contact hypersensitivity* q.v., has an immunological basis.

contact hypersensitivity *Hypersensitivity* reaction of any type provoked in the skin by contact with chemical substances which act as *antigens* or *haptens*. Many cases of *contact dermatitis* are due either to *immediate hypersensitivity* (*histamine* release), e.g. sensitivity to fish skin oils in the fish processing industry or *delayed-type hypersensitivity* (*cell-mediated immunity*), e.g. sensitivity to nickel in wrist watch cases.

convalescent serum A sample of *serum* collected from a patient about three weeks after the onset of a disease. If the *titre* of *antibody* against a microorganism is found to be significantly higher than in a serum specimen collected in the early acute phase of the illness this is considered to indicate infection with that microorganism. A significant rise is taken to be at least fourfold in virus diseases but greater than this in suspected Gram negative bacterial infection due to the possibility of an *anamnestic response*.

conventional animals (holoxenic) All experimental animals other than those that have been reared under *gnotobiotic, germ free* or 'specific pathogen-free' conditions. Currently most small experimental animals (esp. rats and mice) are reared under specific pathogen-free conditions. Whether or not they remain pathogen-free whilst under experiment depends on the maintenance of a *barrier* to infection by the specified organisms. The disparities that arise may result in inconsistency of *immune responses* in the animals when used.

conventional B lymphocyte The common form of *B lymphocyte* in man after infancy. It is *CD5* negative. Term used in contrast to *B-1 lymphocyte* q.v.

Coombs' test See *antiglobulin test*.

cooperation See *T–B cell cooperation*.

coprecipitation The precipitation of soluble immune complexes (see *soluble* *complex*) by the addition of a *secondary antibody* or *protein A*. The second antibody may be directed against the *antigen* or it may be an anti *immunoglobulin*. Commonly used in assays for radiolabelled antigen at very low concentration by the addition of excess antibody, which forms soluble complexes, followed by anti immunoglobulin or protein A.

Corynebacterium parvum Name given to a group of bacteria (rarely pathogenic) which actually belong to the genus *Propionibacterium*. They have *immunopotentiating* effects especially as activators of *macrophages*, and have been used experimentally as immunological *adjuvants*. Strictly speaking, should be grouped as anaerobic coryneform bacteria.

costimulatory molecules Cell surface molecules other than the antigen receptor (*TCR* or *membrane immunoglobulin*) or its ligand (e.g. the *major histocompatibility complex*–antigenic peptide complex) that are required for an efficient response of *lymphocytes* to *antigen*. Such molecules on *T cells* include *CD4* or *CD8*, *CD2*, adhesion molecules, *CD28* (binding to *CD80* on *accessory cells*) or, on *B cells*, *CD40* binding to its T cell ligand (*CD40L*). Antigen binding without costimulation may lead to *anergy* rather than to an *immune response*. Some costimulatory molecules (e.g. CD40 on B cells) may be necessary to rescue lymphocytes from *apoptosis*, e.g. for *positive selection*.

counter current immunoelectrophoresis (CIE) A rapid *precipitin test* in which sensitivity is increased by causing the reactants (*antigen* and *antibody*) to be brought together by an electric current. Cf. *double diffusion test*.

cowpox A virus disease first described by Jenner that causes vesicular eruptions on the teats of cows. The virus is transferable to man in whom it produces lesions similar to those that follow primary vaccination (see *smallpox vaccination*) and gives protection against smallpox (see *variola*). The virus closely resembles *vaccinia* virus except

that it produces haemorrhagic pocks on the chorio-allantoic membrane of the chick embryo.

CR1 (complement receptor 1; CD35) A *Type I transmembrane protein* of the *SCR superfamily*. The extracellular domain consists of 30 short consensus repeats. Found on human *neutrophil leucocytes, mononuclear phagocytes, B lymphocytes, Langerhans cells, follicular dendritic cells,* and glomerular endothelial cells. Binds *C3b* and C4b (see *C4*). Acts as an opsonic receptor (see *opsonin*) for *phagocytosis* of *complement*-coated particles and *immune complexes* and activates a microbicidal metabolic burst following phagocytosis. Also accelerates decay of *C3 convertase* and is a cofactor for *Factor I* mediated cleavage of C3b. See Figure C3.

CR2 (CD21) A *Type I transmembrane protein* of the *SCR superfamily*. The extracellular domain consists of 15 or 16 short consensus repeats. Found chiefly on human mature *B lymphocytes* and *follicular dendritic cells*. Binds C3d (a cleavage product of *C3b*) and also the Epstein–Barr virus and binding regulates B lymphocyte activation and proliferation. Also binds to *CD23*.

CR3 (CD11b) See *CD11* and *CD18*. The integrin α chain (see *integrin superfamily*) of *CD11b*/CD18 and a major *leucocyte*-adhesion molecule. Also binds *iC3b* and thereby has an important role in opsonic *phagocytosis* (see *opsonization*) and bacterial killing. Expression on phagocytic cells is upregulated by inflammatory mediators.

CR4 (CD11c) See *CD11* and *CD18*. The integrin α chain (see *integrin superfamily*) of *CD11c*/CD18 (p150,95). Also binds *iC3b* and therefore can function as an *opsonin*.

CREG See *cross reactive group*.

cross absorption *Absorption* of *antigens* or *antibodies* using cross reacting antibodies or cross reacting antigens.

cross matching (1) A procedure used for selecting blood for transfusion by establishing compatibility between donor and recipient in respect of the *ABO blood group system* and *Rhesus blood group system* and other blood groups as appropriate, usually by testing the compatibility of the recipient's serum with donor cells using *haemagglutination* and an *antiglobulin test*. (2) A procedure for selecting a potentially compatible organ or *bone marrow* donor for transplantation. The procedure consists of testing the recipient's serum against donor peripheral blood *T lymphocytes* and *B lymphocytes*. For *HLA histocompatibility system* antigens, this is usually undertaken as a *complement*-dependent lymphocytotoxic test (see *cytotoxicity tests*) using viability stains (e.g. ethidium bromide and acridine orange) or *flow cytometry* (see *dye exclusion test*).

cross reacting antibody *Antibody* capable of binding to an *antigen* which did not specifically stimulate its production. Depending on the presence and distribution of epitopes this cross reaction may not be as strong as the reaction of the antibody with its own antigen although in some cases it is stronger. Cf. *cross reacting antigen* and see *heteroclitic antibody*.

cross reacting antigen (1) *Antigen* capable of binding to *antibody* produced in response to a different antigen. May cross react due to sharing of epitopes by the two antigens or because the epitopes of each, although not identical, are closely enough related stereochemically to combine with antibody against one of them. (2) Antigen of identical structure in two strains of bacteria, so that antibody produced against one strain will react with the other.

cross reactive group (CREG) Term used specifically of a group of *antigens* of the *major histocompatibility complex* that share the same, or similar, *epitope* as determined by *histocompatibility testing*, e.g. the *HLA histocompatibility system* antigens A1, A1O and A11 share a cross reactive epitope as do A9, A25, A32 and Bw4, and again Cw4 and Cw6 thus forming three distinct types of cross reactive groups. See also *private determinant, public determinant*.

cross sensitivity *Hypersensitivity* to one substance produced by priming (see *primed*) with another substance which bears cross reacting *antigens*.

cross tolerance *Immunological tolerance* against an *antigen* or tissue produced by contact with a different antigen or tissue which bears *cross reacting antigens*.

CRP See *C reactive protein*.

cryoglobulin *Globulin* especially *IgG* or *IgM* which precipitates spontaneously when *serum* is cooled below 37°C and redissolves on warming. Does not occur in normal serum. Cryoglobulinaemia may occur in association with *myelomatosis, macroglobulinaemia, lymphoma* and systemic lupus erythematosus (*SLE*). Characterized by peripheral vascular occlusion (Raynaud's phenomenon) and purpura of the extremities.

CSF See *colony stimulating factors*.

CSF-1 See *M-CSF*.

CTL See *cytotoxic T lymphocyte*.

CTLA-4 A *Type 1 transmembrane protein* of the *Ig superfamily*. Found on activated *T cells* and binds to *CD80* on *B cells* and other *accessory cells*. It is similar in structure, function, chromosomal location and gene arrangement to *CD28*, q.v.

Cunningham plaque technique *Plaque-forming cell assay* carried out in a monolayer of red cells formed between a slide and coverslip, without agar.

cutaneous basophil hypersensitivity A response of the *Jones–Mote reaction* type. A modified *delayed-type hypersensitivity* reaction elicited by inoculation with *PPD*. Demonstrable in guinea pigs, it follows the same time course as the classical delayed-type hypersensitivity reaction but *histamine* levels are increased at the site of inoculation, which lacks fibrin and is less indurated. 20–60% of the infiltrating *inflammatory cells* are *basophil leucocytes*.

cutaneous sensitization Provocation of *hypersensitivity* by cutaneous contact with *antigen*.

cyclophilin Cyclophilins are intracellular proteins which bind cyclosporin (e.g. *cyclosporin A*). The cyclosporin–cyclophilin complex binds to, and inhibits the function of, *calcineurin* q.v. in *T cells*, thus inducing *immunosuppression*. Cyclophilins and *FKBPs* are known collectively as immunophilins.

cyclophosphamide A potent alkylating anti-cancer drug with a place in routine chemotherapy often in combination with other drugs. Though *immunosuppressive*, it does not rival azathioprine or *cyclosporin A* (q.v.) because of *bone marrow* depression. Experimentally it inhibits *lymphocyte* division and *B lymphocytes* are preferentially affected.

cyclosporin A (CyA®) A cyclic 11 amino acid peptide with *immunosuppressive* and antifungal properties. It is widely used in clinical organ and *bone marrow* transplantation. It acts predominantly on *helper T lymphocytes* where it blocks activation early in the G1 phase of growth and selectively impairs *cytokine* (particularly *IL-2*) production through the inhibition of *calcineurin* phosphatase activity within the *T cell* (see also *cyclophilin*, *FK506*). CyA® is nephrotoxic and causes hirsutism and gum hyperplasia.

cytokine receptor superfamily A family of *Type I transmembrane proteins*, many of which are *receptors* for *cytokines* or for haemopoietic growth factors or for hormones. Also known as the haemopoietic growth factor receptor superfamily or the haemopoietin superfamily. They share a 100-residue 'cytokine receptor' *domain* and a domain also found in fibronectin (the fibronectin Type III superfamily domains), and some also contain *Ig superfamily* domains. In this superfamily are the receptors for *G-CSF*, *GM-CSF*, *IL-2* (β-chain), *IL-3*, *IL-4*, *IL-5* and *IL-6*.

cytokines Generic name for proteins made and secreted by cells, which act as intercellular mediators with effects on growth, differentiation, activation, etc. of the same or other cells. Cytokines are important non-*antigen*-specific effector molecules in many immune and inflammatory responses. *Lymphocytes* are an important source of cytokines (lymphokines, e.g. *IL-2*, *IL-4*, *IFN-γ*) and their release is often stimulated following contact with antigen. Cytokines released by *mononuclear phagocytes* (e.g. *IL-1*, *TNF-α*) are known as monokines. Release of these is often stimulated by inflammatory signals or signals resulting from lymphocyte activation in an *immune response*. It should be noted that cytokines have numerous functions outside the immune system, e.g. in developmental biology.

cytolytic T lymphocyte See *cytotoxic T lymphocyte*.

cytotoxic T lymphocyte (CTL; cytolytic T lymphocyte; Tc; T_{CTX}) Effector *T lymphocyte* subset (usually *CD8+*, *class I MHC antigen* restricted) which directly lyses target cells. Cytotoxic T lymphocytes kill virus-infected cells provided that the latter carry *syngeneic* class I MHC antigens (see *MHC restriction*). Two major mechanisms are used for killing: (a) release of *perforins*, and (b) cytotoxic T lymphocyte-membrane *Fas* ligand binds to Fas on target cells thus inducing *apoptosis* in the latter.

cytotoxicity tests Tests of cell killing. For example, following incubation of cells either with specific *antibody* and *complement*, or with *cytotoxic T lymphocytes* which have been *primed* against *antigens* on the cell surface, the cells are damaged as a result of an immune reaction against their surface antigens. Loss of viability can then be demonstrated by a *dye exclusion test* q.v. Cytotoxicity tests are used in *histocompatibility testing* (HLA typing) in which sera against specific HLA molecules (see *HLA histocompatibility system*) will cause complement-mediated lysis when added to *lymphocytes* which express the HLA type against which the antibodies in the test serum are directed.

D

D exon A short sequence of DNA coding for part of the third *hypervariable region* of the *heavy chain*, found on the 5′ side of the *J exons* but separated from them by an *intron*. At least five D (diversity) exons are associated with the human μ *constant region* gene and two with the human T cell receptor (*TCR*) β and δ chain gene loci. During the differentiation of a *stem cell* to a *lymphocyte* a D exon is translocated to the position immediately 5′ to one of the J exons to which it becomes attached. A V exon with its associated Lp exon, then translocates to the position 5′ to the combined D–J exon to form a continuous V–D–J sequence coding for the entire *variable region*. See Figures I4 and I5.

D-gene See *D exon*.

DAF See *decay accelerating factor*.

dander antigen A mixture of materials continually being shed from the skin surface. Includes desquamated epithelial cells, hair fragments, microorganisms and other materials entrained in the sebum and sweat. Cat dander remains airborne for long periods and is strongly implicated as a cause of *immediate hypersensitivity* reactions, mainly *asthma*, in atopic persons (see *atopy*). Occupational asthma among veterinary surgeons and workers with laboratory animals can be caused by a wide variety of animal danders. In the case of the latter a mask supplying filtered air to the eyes, nose and mouth may be necessary for protection.

dark zone See *germinal centre*.

decay accelerating factor (DAF; CD55) This control protein of the *complement* system is a *GPI anchor*-linked membrane protein (70 kD) of the *SCR superfamily* found on erythrocytes, platelets,

monocytes, *neutrophil leucocytes*, and other granulocytes. DAF inhibits the formation of convertase (see *C4*) on the cell surface by interacting with bound *C3b* or C4b. It is also reported to accelerate the decay of surface-bound convertases. This controls spontaneous self lysis. Lacking in *paroxysmal nocturnal haemoglobinuria* (q.v.).

decomplementation Removal of haemolytic activity of *complement* from *serum* by *heat inactivation, cobra venom* factor, *zymosan, immune complexes*, etc. or removal of complement activity from whole animals by treatment with such agents.

defensin Defensins are a family of small disulphide-bonded peptides (29–34 residues) which are arginine-rich and therefore positively charged. They constitute about 30% of the granule-associated protein in *neutrophil leucocytes* and are also found in *macrophages*. They bind to membranes of bacteria and fungi, increase membrane permeability, and kill the target microorganisms.

delayed cell-mediated reaction Reaction of *cell-mediated immunity*. See also *delayed-type hypersensitivity*.

delayed cutaneous reaction An erythematous, oedematous, reaction seen maximally in the skin 48 hours after application of a sensitizing agent (see *sensitization*). The reaction is mainly *lymphocyte* mediated, but requires the ability to mount an inflammatory response, e.g. presence of *inflammatory cells* and release of *vascular permeability factors*, for full expression.

delayed hypersensitivity See *delayed-type hypersensitivity*.

delayed-type hypersensitivity (DTH; delayed hypersensitivity) *Hypersensi-*

tivity state mediated by primed *T lymphocytes*. The lesions, in which *lymphocytes* and *macrophages* are usually prominent, do not appear until about 24 hours after *challenge* of a *primed* subject with *antigen*, e.g. by intradermal inoculation. Cf. *immediate hypersensitivity* and *Arthus reaction*. The ability to react in this way can be transferred to another animal only with lymphocytes (from *lymph node, spleen*, etc.) and is a manifestation of *cell-mediated immunity* q.v. Cytokines made by T_H1 *cells* such as *IL-2* and *IFN-γ*, are believed to play a prominent role in the development of the lesion.

dendritic cell The dendritic cells are a system of cells of stellate or dendritic morphology which are constitutively strongly *class II MHC antigen* positive and are important *accessory cells*, essential for *primary immune responses*. Originally derived from *bone marrow*, they are found throughout the body both in sites of contact with *antigen* (skin *Langerhans cells*, dendritic cells in gut, lung, etc.), and in *peripheral lymphoid organs*. The peripherally sited dendritic cells may be immature, bear *Fc receptors* and *C3b receptors* and are capable of *antigen processing* and *antigen presentation*. On contact with antigen, these migrate to *lymphoid tissues*, lose the above receptors, no longer process antigen, but are potent *antigen-presenting cells*. Note that the *follicular dendritic cells* (q.v.) found in germinal centres are unrelated to the cells described above and are not bone marrow derived.

density gradient centrifugation A method for separating cells or large molecules, e.g. proteins, nucleic acids, of different types by centrifugation through a density gradient. When used to separate cells, the medium must be incapable of penetrating the cell membrane, e.g. *Percoll*® (colloidal silica), Ficoll-Hypaque®. Centrifugation may be: (a) Isokinetic (velocity sedimentation), in which the cells or molecules separate according to size as they move through the gradient. This is not now commonly used. (b) Isopyknic (equilibrium sedimentation), in which the cells or molecules sediment through the gradient until they reach a

point at which their specific gravity is equal to that of the medium. They therefore separate into bands of differing density. Widely used for the isolation of *lymphocytes*, and of *stem cells* from *bone marrow*.

Dermatophagoides pteronyssinus A mite present in house dust. *Antigens* derived from the mite, mainly proteases from its faecal pellets, are potent *allergens* in stimulating the production of *IgE* antibody in atopic persons (see *atopy*). These allergens are the most common cause of *asthma* in the UK. See also *house dust allergy*.

desensitization See *hyposensitization*.

despecification Treatment of heterologous therapeutic *antisera* (e.g. *diphtheria antitoxin* made in horses) to reduce their *antigenicity*, so that they are less likely to cause *hypersensitivity* reactions. Achieved by separating the *immunoglobulin* fraction which is then subjected to *pepsin digestion* to remove the *Fc fragment* but retain the *antigen*-specific $F(ab')_2$ *fragment*.

determinant See *epitope*.

dextrans In immunological context these substances are *mitogens* for *B lymphocytes* of mice activating the cells at a primitive stage of differentiation. Chemically they are polysaccharides made up of glucose residues and some are *thymus independent antigens* (*TI-2 antigens*). See also *polyclonal activators*.

Di George's syndrome Failure of development of the parathyroids and *thymus* due to intrauterine damage to the third and fourth pharyngeal pouches. There is a defect manifest in infancy of *cell-mediated immunity* with low levels of circulating *T lymphocytes*, together with hypocalcaemia and tetany, and congenital heart defects. See *thymic hypoplasia*.

dialysis The use of semipermeable membranes to separate substances of differing molecular weights in solution.

Equilibrium dialysis (q.v.) is used for the measurement of antibody *affinity*.

diphtheria antitoxin Antibody against the *exotoxin* of *Corynebacterium diphtheriae* produced by hyperimmunizing horses with *diphtheria toxoid*.

diphtheria toxoid *Toxoid* prepared by formalin treatment of the *exotoxin* of *Corynebacterium diphtheriae* thus destroying its toxic activity. Used prophylactically for *active immunization* against diphtheria.

direct immunofluorescence (single layer immunofluorescence technique). *Immunofluorescence* technique in which *antigen* is detected with a single layer of *fluorochrome*-conjugated *antibody* or, less commonly, where antibody is detected with a single layer of fluorochrome-conjugated antigen. See Figure D1.

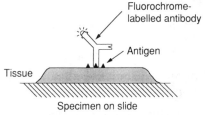

Figure D1. Direct immunofluorescence technique.

disodium cromoglycate (DSCG) A drug of considerable prophylactic value in certain illnesses due to *immediate hypersensitivity* (*type I hypersensitivity reactions*) notably *asthma*. Usually administered by inhalation but can also be given orally and topically to eyes and nose. Its action is unknown although several mechanisms, viz. stabilization of *mast cell* membranes, bridging of *IgE* molecules (and exclusion of *antigen* bridging) on mast cells, or enzyme–substrate chelation, have been suggested.

dissociation constant See K_d and also *association constant*.

diversity See *repertoire* and *D exon*.

domain Sequence of a protein or peptide that forms a discrete structural unit, e.g.

the *constant regions* and *variable regions* of *immunoglobulins*. Protein superfamilies comprise groups of proteins all of which contain domains with related tertiary structures, though the primary sequences within these domains may be different. The different superfamilies are defined on the basis of their content of such domains. See *homology region*.

Donath–Landsteiner antibody Haemolytic *antibody* in *paroxysmal cold haemoglobinuria*. Binds at low temperature to the P blood group antigens on the patient's own red cells or on normal erythrocytes and causes *haemolysis* on warming the cells.

dot blotting (dot immunoblotting) A technique for the rapid detection of an *antigen* in a fluid. The antigen solution is spotted on to a membrane, usually nitrocellulose, dried and detected by incubation with a *primary antibody* followed by a labelled *secondary antibody*, as in *immunoblotting*. The label can be any of the detection systems used in immunoblotting but a radioisotope label or enzyme-conjugated second antibody are the most popular. Dot blotting is essentially qualitative or semi quantitative but can be used quantitatively by densitometry. Slot blotting is essentially identical to dot blotting except that a template is used to apply the sample as a uniform band (or slot) which makes quantification by densitometry easier.

double diffusion test A *gel diffusion test* in which solutions of *antigen* and of *antibody* diffuse towards one another to form lines of *precipitation*. Used to analyse purity of antigens and antibodies in solutions and to analyse the antigenic relationships of different substances with one another. See *Ouchterlony test, reaction of identity, reaction of partial identity, reaction of non-identity, spur*.

double labelling Any technique in which two reagents, most commonly *antibodies*, are labelled with different markers, so that both can be detected in the same preparation. Most frequently used in *immunofluorescence* techniques where, for example, one antibody, e.g.

anti *CD3*, is labelled green with *FITC*, and another, e.g. anti *CD19*, is labelled red with *phycoerythrin*. Thus *T cells* (CD3+) stain green and *B cells* (CD19+) stain red. This is the basis for current evaluation of T and B cells numbers by *flow cytometry* or fluorescence microscopy and there are numerous other applications.

double layer immunofluorescence An *indirect immunofluorescence* technique in which *antigen* is detected with unlabelled *primary antibody* followed by a *fluorochrome*-labelled *secondary antibody* reactive against the primary antibody in the first layer. More sensitive than *direct immunofluorescence* due to a multiplication effect as more sites for combination are available. The same labelled secondary antibody can also be used in several systems, i.e. in diagnosis of disease it can reveal whether there are *antibodies* in a patient's serum which have become attached to test antigens. See Figure I6.

double-negative thymocytes Immature *thymocytes* which express neither *CD4* nor *CD8*.

double-positive thymocytes *Thymocytes* which have differentiated from the *double-negative thymocyte* phenotype and which express both *CD4* and *CD8*. This transition occurs once the cells begin to make *TCR* β chains. Further maturation, and expression of TCR α chains, are followed by *positive selection* and *negative selection* of *antigen*-reactive TCR+, single-positive (CD4+ or CD8+), *T cells*.

doubling dilution Method of preparing serial dilutions for use in serological tests. To dilute a reagent for titration, one volume of it is added to one volume of saline in a tube. The contents are mixed and one volume is taken and added to one volume of saline in a second tube. The procedure is repeated to the end of a row of tubes so that the dilution of reagent in each tube is double that in the previous one, i.e. 1 in 2, 1 in 4, 1 in 8, 1 in 16, etc.

drug allergy *Hypersensitivity* to drugs. May be of any type (See *type I, II, III* and *IV hypersensitivity reactions*), systemic, or local depending on route of administration. Skin lesions are frequently seen (*contact dermatitis, eczema*, urticaria, etc.). Many drugs act as *antigens* or *haptens* and hypersensitivity reactions to a huge list of them have been reported. For example see *penicillin hypersensitivity*.

DTH See *delayed-type hypersensitivity*.

DTH T cell See T_{DTH} *lymphocyte*.

Duncan's syndrome See *X-linked lymphoproliferative syndrome*.

dye exclusion test *In vitro* test for viability of cells. Living cells exclude membrane-impermeable dyes such as trypan blue or eosin, whereas dead cells take them up and become stained. Can also be used quantitatively with fluorescent dyes which can be measured using *flow cytometry*. Note: the dye exclusion test may not detect cells that die by *apoptosis*, in which the cell membrane initially remains intact. See also *cytotoxicity tests*.

E

E-rosette forming cell A *lymphocyte* that forms spontaneous *rosettes* with sheep erythrocytes. The sheep erythrocytes bind to the *T cell*-specific marker *CD2* and E-rosette formation is presently accepted as a T lymphocyte marker in man and most mammals. The method can be improved by pretreating the erythrocytes with AET (see *AET rosette test*) or neuraminidase. Do not confuse E-rosette forming cells with *EAC–rosette forming cells* q.v.

E-selectin See *selectins*.

EA Symbol for an erythrocyte with *antibody* bound to its surface membrane, as in 'EA rosetting', a method for measuring the activity of *Fc receptors*.

EAC Abbreviation used in *complement* studies where E is erythrocyte (usually a sheep red blood cell), A is anti sheep red blood cell *antibody* bound to the surface membrane and C is complement. The sequence of fixation of individual complement components may then follow thus, EAC1423, etc.

EAC–rosette forming cell A cell that forms rosettes with sheep erythrocytes in the presence of anti sheep red blood cell *antibody* (A) and *complement* (C). Rosetting takes place by binding of the red cells to *C3b receptors (CR1)*. EAC rosette formation has been used as a *B lymphocyte* marker. Phagocytic cells (see *phagocyte*) possess C3b receptors (CR1, *CR3* and *CR4*) and can therefore also form EAC rosettes.

EAE See *experimental allergic encephalomyelitis*.

ECF-A (eosinophil chemotactic factors of *anaphylaxis*) Chemotactic factors (see *chemotaxis*) for *eosinophil leucocytes* that are released from *mast cells* when *IgE* antibody bound to them reacts with *antigen*.

eczema Itching, inflammatory, non-contagious skin eruption usually irregular in distribution and character so that papules, vesicles and pustules may be present together with oedema, scaling or exudation. Occurs in highly *atopic* persons (atopic dermatitis) or may follow ingestion or local applications of haptenic drugs (see *hapten*) so that many cases are probably manifestations of *hypersensitivity* of various types. Common in children, usually under 2 years and associated with foods mainly eggs and groundnuts (peanuts). These children may later develop *asthma* q.v.

ED$_{50}$ The 50% effective dose.

education Process by which a pool of *receptor*-bearing *T lymphocytes* or *B lymphocytes* which do not recognize self *antigens*, but which are fully responsive to foreign antigens, is generated.

effector cell A cell that performs defined effector functions in *immunity*[1] either directly or as a result of signals from *antigen*-reactive *lymphocytes*. *Effector lymphocytes, neutrophil leucocytes, eosinophil leucocytes, mast cells,* and *macrophages* all perform effector functions, e.g. *phagocytosis*, microbial killing, mediator release, *cytokine* release and others.

effector lymphocyte Lymphocyte which as a result of antigen-dependent differentiation has a direct functional role in the *immune response*. E.g. *cytotoxic T lymphocyte, helper T lymphocyte, plasma cell*.

Ehrlich's side chain theory An early *selective theory of antibody production* proposed by Paul Ehrlich in 1900. He suggested that cells carried *receptor* groups with 'haptophore' side chains on their surfaces. On contact with antigen the side chains combined with it and the receptors were then thrown off the cell to be replaced by new ones. Antibody consisted of such receptors that had been thrown off into the circulation.

ELAM-1 See *selectins*.

elicited macrophage *Macrophage* present at a site as a result of an eliciting stimulus. Contrast with the *resident macrophage*.

ELISA (enzyme-linked immunosorbent assay) An immunoassay in which *antigen* or *antibody* is detected by the binding of an enzyme coupled to either *antibody* specific for the *antigen* or anti *immunoglobulin*. The principle of the technique is similar to that of the sandwich and double-layer variations of *indirect immunofluorescence* (see Figure I6) except that the fluorochrome is replaced by an enzyme. To detect antibody: antigen is adsorbed on to the surface of wells, plastic test tubes or beads followed by the test sample. After washing away unbound material any antigen–antibody complexes formed when the sample was applied are detected by the application of an anti immunoglobulin conjugated to an enzyme. When this reacts with its substrate a coloured product results which may be measured spectrophotometrically. Commonly used enzymes are horseradish peroxidase and alkaline phosphatase and the colour produced is proportional in intensity to the concentration of antibody being measured. To detect antigen: its specific antibody is bound to the well surface and after application of the sample any antigen in it that has combined with the antibody is detected by a second antibody from a different species. The attachment of this to the antigen is demonstrated by an enzyme-conjugated anti immunoglobulin in the same way as for the antibody.

ELISPOT assay A technique for measurement of the number of *B cells* secreting specific *antibody*. *Antigen* is coated on to a nitrocellulose membrane which forms the base of a multi-well plate. A cell suspension is incubated in the wells and antibody secreted by individual cells diffuses radially outwards and binds to the antigen on the membrane in a small circular area around the cell. The cells are then washed off and the bound antibody detected by a *secondary antibody*, an enzyme conjugated anti *immunoglobulin*. Horseradish peroxidase or alkaline phosphatase are the enzymes generally used and colour is developed using a chromogenic substrate that is converted to an insoluble coloured product. This precipitates on the membrane as a coloured spot and the number of spots is proportional to the number of antibody-secreting cells. The ELISPOT assay has replaced the earlier Jerne and Cunningham *plaque-forming cell assays* due to its greater reliability, versatility, and the ease with which the class of antibody secreted by individual cells can be determined by using *immunoglobulin class* specific secondary antibodies. The ELISPOT assay can, in principle, be adapted to enumerate cells secreting any molecule using a *sandwich technique*. In place of antigen, the membrane is coated with antibody specific for the molecule of interest. Spots are developed using a second antibody against the same molecule. This adaptation has been used to enumerate cells secreting *cytokines*.

ellipsoids Fusiform structures that surround the capillaries at the terminations of the penicillar arterioles of the *spleen* where these enter the *red pulp*. They consist of a sheath of high (or cuboidal) endothelial cells. If carbon or other particles are experimentally injected into the blood stream it is at this sheath that the most active *phagocytosis* takes place; *macrophages* containing the carbon are seen ringing the ellipsoids. Ellipsoids are prominent in the spleens of birds, pigs, horses and cats, but are difficult to distinguish in man and are absent in rodents.

emperipolesis The apparent penetration of *lymphocytes* into (and their continuous movement within) other cells as monitored by time-lapse cinematography. It is doubtful whether it actually occurs.

ENAs (extractable nuclear antigens) Nuclear and cytoplasmic *antigens* which are readily extractable in buffer. Many of these antigens are now described against which patients with connective tissue disease make *auto-antibodies*. They are detected by *counter current immunoelectrophoresis, ELISA,* or *immunoblotting*. Of greatest clinical importance are antibodies to Ro, La, Sm, RNP, Scl-70 and Jo-1.

encapsulation *Leucocyte* response to foreign objects too large to be ingested. In invertebrates, such as molluscs, annelids and arthropods, this is the typical *immune response*. The object is walled off by a many-layered capsule of flattened leucocytes (*haemocytes* or *coelomocytes*); in arthropods this may also be associated with production of melanin around the object. Similar responses are also seen in vertebrate tissues, e.g. to foreign bodies or to metazoan parasites. These objects become surrounded by *macrophages* and other leucocytes, which form a *granuloma*, and later by fibroblasts. The end result is a fibrous capsule.

encephalitogenic factors Substances present in extracts of brain which, when injected together with *complete Freund's adjuvant*, are capable of eliciting *experimental allergic encephalomyelitis* in experimental animals. A basic protein resembling histone, associated with myelin (myelin basic protein), is the most important of these.

end cell A cell that is the end product of maturation and is no longer capable of maturing further, e.g. the mature *plasma cell* is an end cell in the *lymphoid cell series*.

end point The highest dilution to which an *antiserum* or *antibody* solution can be carried, yet still show a detectable reaction with *antigen*, thus giving the *titre* q.v.

endocytosis Internalization of particles or fluid by cells by enclosure in a 'pit' of invaginated plasma membrane followed by closure of the pit to form an intracellular vesicle containing the ingested material. Ingestion of particles is called *phagocytosis*; ingestion of fluid, pinocytosis. Two forms of endocytosis are recognized; receptor-mediated endocytosis and fluid-phase endocytosis. In receptor-mediated endocytosis, particles or molecules bound to membrane *receptors* are internalized in clathrin-coated vesicles (clathrin is a protein shaped like a three-legged structure which polymerizes to form a basket-like network round the vesicle). Fluid-phase endocytosis, which occurs more slowly, is internalization of fluid and of molecules dissolved in it, without a requirement for receptors, into vesicles that may or may not be clathrin-coated. After internalization, coated vesicles lose their clathrin and fuse with other vesicles to form endosomes, the contents of which become acidified. Endosomes may fuse with *lysosomes* in which case their contents are digested or, in *antigen processing* they may be the site of peptidebinding to *class II MHC antigens* and be recycled subsequently to the plasma membrane. *Macrophages* constitutively have a high rate of fluid phase endocytosis such that the entire plasma membrane is internalized every 30 minutes and recycled back to the cell surface.

endoplasmic reticulum A tubular cytoplasmic structure consisting of paired (parallel) membranes attached to the nuclear membrane. Present in all cells, it is most highly developed in protein-secreting cells where it is called rough-surfaced endoplasmic reticulum (RER) because of the numerous ribosomes attached to it. RER is prominent in protein-secreting cells such as *plasma cells* which secrete *immunoglobulins*.

endotoxin Classically, a bacteriologist's term for toxins that are only released on the death of the bacterial cell, as opposed to the diffusible *exotoxins* (q.v.) that are produced by living bacteria. Nowadays, however, the term is used almost exclusively as a synonym for the *lipopolysaccharides* q.v. of Gram negative bacteria. It should be noted, however, that the term is descriptive only and that no one substance 'endotoxin' exists.

endotoxin shock Syndrome following administration of *lipopolysaccharide* (LPS) in man or experimental animals, or following infection with *endotoxin*-producing bacteria. Mice and rabbits are killed by small doses of LPS (30 μg/kg) and 0.02 μg/kg is sufficient to cause fever in man (typically seen following administration of typhoid vaccine). Characterized by prostration and hypotension, fever and leucopenia. A local or general *Shwartzman reaction* with renal cortical necrosis is seen in severe cases. High levels of *TNF-α* and *IL-1* are present and may mediate much of the pathology. See also *septic shock*.

enhancement See *immunological enhancement*.

enzyme labelling Methods for tracing *antibodies* or *antigens* in tissue sections by binding them chemically to an enzyme and then, by using a colour reagent specific for that enzyme, locating the antibody or antigen. The *peroxidase–anti peroxidase* (PAP) and alkaline phosphatase/anti alkaline phosphatase (*APAAP*) techniques are examples of such methods. Principle similar to that used in *immunofluorescence* and *autoradiography*. See also *ELISA*.

enzyme-linked immunosorbent assay See *ELISA*.

eosinophil leucocyte A *granulocyte* found in normal blood (40–440 cells/mm^3 in man, i.e. up to 6% of total white cells), characterized by a bilobed nucleus and large, eosinophilic, cytoplasmic granules rich in cationic proteins. The electron-dense core of the granule contains major basic protein (MBP). Other granule constituents include eosinophil cationic protein, eosinophil-derived neurotoxin and eosinophil peroxidase. Development of eosinophils in the *bone marrow* is separate from that of other granulocytes, e.g. *neutrophil leucocytes*, and is regulated by *cytokines*, e.g. *IL-5*, *IL-3* and *GM-CSF*. IL-5 also stimulates functions of mature eosinophils, enhances their sur-

vival and increases their cytotoxicity. Eosinophils have *Fc receptors* and *C3b receptors* but are not strongly *phagocytic*. Rather they respond to large targets, e.g. metazoan parasites, by secretion and release of granule contents. They are prominent in the lesions of *immediate hypersensitivity*, e.g. *asthma*, and in metazoan parasitic infections, and there is frequently a blood *eosinophilia* associated with these conditions.

eosinophilia Increase in numbers of *eosinophil leucocytes* q.v. especially in blood, above physiological levels. Particularly associated with *immediate hypersensitivity* reactions and responses to nematode worm infections.

epithelioid cell A morphologically compressed *macrophage* with pale pink cytoplasm, indistinct cell membrane and large pale oval nucleus (H & E stain) found in *granulomata* such as those that occur in tuberculosis.

epitope The region on an *antigen* molecule to which *antibody* or the *TCR* (T cell receptor) binds specifically. Epitopes are also known as 'antigenic determinants'. B cell epitopes on protein antigens are of variable size comprising up to about 20 amino acids. Antibodies bind in a more or less exact three-dimensional fit with an epitope. This may be formed from residues on different regions of a protein antigen molecule which, in the native state, are closely apposed due to protein folding. Thus the three-dimensional structure of the protein molecule may be essential for antibody binding. Epitopes recognized by *T cells* are peptide fragments which have been processed by an *accessory cell* and presented in the cleft of a *class I MHC antigen* or *class II MHC antigen* molecule, thus the T cell recognizes the peptide bound to *syngeneic* MHC. Since a continuous primary sequence is necessary for T cell recognition but not for antibody recognition, the epitopes recognized on the same protein molecule by each are different. Also a single protein antigen may carry several different epitopes. Polysaccharide epitopes may consist of repeating unit structures. New epitopes can be created on antigen molecules by covalent linking of *haptens*.

epitype A family of related *epitopes* q.v.

equilibrium dialysis A technique used to study the *primary interaction* between a *hapten* and *antibody* to it. A container is divided into two parts by a cellophane *dialysis* membrane impermeable to the antibody but not to the hapten. The antibody is placed on one side of this and the hapten on the other. When equilibrium has been reached, the hapten has passed through the membrane so that equal numbers of free hapten molecules are present on each side. Also, on the antibody side additional hapten is present which is bound to the antibody. By using a radioactively labelled hapten and determining the ratio of bound to free hapten the average intrinsic *association constant* of the hapten–antibody interaction can be determined.

equivalence See *optimal proportions*.

erythroblastosis fetalis A disease of the human fetus resulting from maternal–fetal *blood group* incompatibility. During pregnancy (especially during labour) fetal erythrocytes escape into the maternal blood stream and may cause the mother to develop *antibody* to *isoantigens* (commonly *Rhesus blood group system* antigens) not present on her own red cells but inherited by the fetus from the father. During a subsequent pregnancy, the antibody, if of *IgG* type, passes through the placenta into the fetal circulation. *Haemolytic anaemia* may then occur if the erythrocytes of this, subsequent, fetus also exhibit the corresponding antigen. Clinical manifestations include stillbirth, generalized oedema (hydrops fetalis), anaemia, jaundice, kernicterus. May be prevented by giving mother *anti-D* within 36 hours after parturition.

η (eta) **chain** A protein that associates with the *TCR/CD3* complex on *T cells*. It is an alternatively spliced variant of the **ζ** (zeta) *chain* (q.v.). The latter usually exists as a homodimer but, in some T cell lines, ζ forms a heterodimer with η.

exon A continuous sequence of DNA within a gene that codes for an amino acid sequence within the gene product, bounded on either side by non-coding regions (*introns*). The *light chain* genes of *immunoglobulins* are composed of exons coding for the *leader peptide* (Lp), *variable region* (V), the third *hypervariable region* (J) and the *constant region* (C). The *heavy chain* gene is composed of Lp, *V exon*, *D exon* (diversity) and *J exon* (joining) together with exons coding for each domain of the constant region (see Figure I5). The genes for the *TCR* and other members of the *Ig superfamily* are similarly constructed of exons coding for separate domains, see Figure T2.

exotoxin Term used of extracellular bacterial toxins that diffuse from living bacterial cells and cause toxic effects in sites that may be remote from the locus of bacterial growth. The classical descriptive terms exotoxin and *endotoxin* are, however, inadequate since toxigenesis and toxin release are dependent on the stage of growth of the bacterial cells and many toxins do not fit into either category. The classical exotoxins are diphtheria toxin and the clostridial toxins, e.g. tetanus toxin. These can be chemically treated to form *toxoids* q.v. and thus be used in immunization. See also *diphtheria toxoid*.

experimental allergic encephalomyelitis *Autoimmune disease* produced in various species of animal by injections of preparations of brain or spinal cord, usually incorporated in *complete Freund's adjuvant* (CFA). Ten days or so after injection an acute encephalomyelitis develops that is characterized by focal perivascular infiltrations with *lymphocytes* and *macrophages*, and usually demyelination. *Antibody* in the *serum* does not correlate closely with the disease, but *delayed type hypersensitivity* may be of importance. Can also be induced by injecting purified myelin basic protein in CFA. See also *encephalitogenic factors*.

experimental allergic neuritis Peripheral neuritis produced in experimental animals by injection of extracts of peripheral nerve in *complete Freund's adjuvant*. An *autoimmune disease*.

experimental allergic thyroiditis *Autoimmune disease* of the thyroid produced by injecting thyroid extract or thyroglobulin in *complete Freund's adjuvant* into experimental animals. Resembles *Hashimoto's thyroiditis* in man.

extractable nuclear antigens See *ENAs*.

extrinsic allergic alveolitis (EAA; also known as hypersensitivity pneumonitis in N. American literature) A restrictive lung disease with constitutional fever and chills (influenza-like symptoms) caused by inhaling organic dusts. The most common syndromes are *bird fancier's lung* and *farmer's lung*. The dusts usually contain particles of about 1 μm diameter which can penetrate and settle in the alveoli, and which carry soluble *antigens*. These particles may also have an *adjuvant* effect since high *titres* of serum *antibody* to the soluble antigen, and raised *immunoglobulin* levels can be measured in sensitized subjects. Broncho-alveolar lavage demonstrates predominantly *lymphocytes* (mainly *CD4* in active disease and *CD8* in chronic disease) and foamy *macrophages* in the alveoli. The interstitium contains an infiltrate mainly of lymphocytes with *granuloma* formation. This gives a characteristic ground-glass appearance on X-ray. The signs and symptoms usually resolve quickly with steroid therapy and antigen avoidance.

F

F₁ hybrid Heterozygote belonging to the first generation derived from crossing genetically dissimilar parents.

Fab fragment Fragment obtained by papain hydrolysis of *immunoglobulin* molecules. The Fab fragment (MW approx. 45 kD) consists of one *light chain* linked to the N-terminal half of the contiguous *heavy chain* (the *Fd fragment*, see Figure I2). Two Fab fragments are obtained from each four chain molecule. Each contains one *antigen-binding site* and so can combine with *antigen* as a *univalent antibody* but cannot form precipitates (see *precipitation*).

F(ab')₂ fragment Fragment obtained by pepsin digestion of *immunoglobulin* molecules (MW approx. 90 kD). The F(ab')₂ fragment consists of that part of the immunoglobulin molecule which is on the N-terminal side of the site of pepsin digestion (see Figure I2) and therefore contains both *Fab fragments* plus the hinge region. It has two *antigen-binding sites*, behaves as divalent *antibody* but does not contain the sites for *complement fixation* and *Fc receptor* binding, both of which are found on the *Fc fragment*.

Facb (fragment antigen and complement binding) Residue of *IgG* molecule remaining after *pFc'* fragment has been removed from the *Fc fragment* portion by action of the enzyme plasmin. Includes all of the molecule except the C_H3 *domain* (see C_H1 etc.).

FACS See *fluorescence activated cell sorter*.

Factor B (C3 proactivator) A component of the *alternative pathway* of *complement* activation. Once complexed with *C3b* it is cleaved by *Factor D* to form the *alternative pathway C3 convertase* (C3bBb). Thus C3b formed by either the *classical complement pathway* or alternative pathway of complement activation can trigger the alternative pathway and initiate a positive feedback amplification mechanism.

Factor D̄ A serine esterase of the *alternative pathway* of *complement* activation. It cleaves *Factor B* when the latter is complexed with *C3b* to form C3bBb from C3bB.

Factor H A glycoprotein that binds to *C3b* and can impair binding of *Factor B* to C3b, accelerate dissociation of Bb from C3b and facilitate conversion of C3b to iC3b by *Factor I*. Thus acts as *complement inhibitor* for the *alternative pathway*.

Factor I (C3b inactivator) A plasma enzyme which cleaves *C3b* to form iC3b. The latter cannot react with *CR1* or participate in *immune cytolysis* or *alternative pathway* activation. Requires *Factor H* as cofactor for its activity on fluid-phase C3b. This cofactor activity can be replaced by CR1.

farmer's lung A syndrome of the *extrinsic allergic alveolitis* (q.v.) type. It is a disease mainly of farmworkers due in most instances to *hypersensitivity* to spores of thermophilic bacteria, mainly *Faenia rectivergula* (*Micropolyspora faeni*) and *Thermoactinomyces vulgaris*; organisms which occur in the dust of mouldy hay. Characterized by attacks of breathlessness and fever a few hours after inhalation of the dust. Can result in diffuse interstitial pneumonitis with heavy cellular infiltration of the alveolar wall, mainly by *monocytes* and *lymphocytes*. May result in pulmonary fibrosis. Precipitating antibodies (see *precipitation*) are present in the *serum* of almost all patients. The disease is probably an example of an **Arthus reaction** (*type III hypersensitivity reaction*) although *delayed-type hypersensitivity* (*type IV hypersensitivity reaction*) may play a part.

Farr test A *radioimmunoassay* technique for measuring specific *antibody* based on the *primary interaction* of antibody with *antigen* in solution. The antibody is allowed to react with radiolabelled antigen or *hapten* and then precipitated with 40% saturated ammonium sulphate. Any antigen or hapten molecules bound to the antibody are precipitated with it while the unbound antigen remains in the supernatant. Not suitable for antigens that are precipitated by ammonium sulphate.

Fas (CD95) A *Type I transmembrane protein* of the *TNFR superfamily* expressed on many cell types including those of the *myeloid cell series* and *lymphoid cell series*. Cross-linking by anti-Fas *antibody* or by the natural Fas ligand induces *apoptosis* of the Fas-bearing cell. Fas is the murine equivalent of human Apo-1.

Fc fragment The crystallizable fragment obtained by papain hydrolysis of *immunoglobulin* molecules. The Fc fragment of human *IgG* has a molecular weight of 50 kD and consists of the C-terminal half of the two *heavy chains* linked by disulphide bonds. It has no *antibody* activity but contains the sites for *complement* and *Fc receptor* binding, placental transmission. and the carbohydrate moiety of the molecule. It also carries some of the *Gm allotype* markers as well as IgG specific and IgG *immunoglobulin subclass* specific *epitopes*. The Fc fragments of other immunoglobulins differ in molecular weight, primary structure and antigenic composition from that of IgG (see Figure I2).

Fc' fragment A fragment produced in small amounts after papain hydrolysis of an *immunoglobulin* molecule, in addition to the *Fc fragment*. It is a noncovalently bonded dimer of the $C_\gamma 3$ *homology region* but without the terminal 13 amino acids, i.e. it is composed of the two $C_H 3$ domains (see $C_H 1$ etc.).

The molecular weight of the dimer is 24 kD (human *IgG*). Present in normal urine in small quantities. Cf. *pFc' fragment*.

Fc receptor *Receptor*, found on the plasma membrane of various cells, that binds the *Fc fragment* of *immunoglobulin*. A number of these receptors have been characterized; details are given in the following three definitions.

Fcα receptor (IgA Fc receptor, FcαR, CD89) A *Type I transmembrane protein* of the *Ig superfamily*. Found chiefly on cells of the *myeloid cell series* (neutrophils and mononuclear phagocytes). Can activate *phagocytosis* and the microbicidal metabolic burst in these cells.

Fcε receptors (IgE Fc receptors, FcεR) (a) FcεRI. A molecular complex comprising an α, a β, and two γ chains. The α chain is a *Type I transmembrane protein* of the *Ig superfamily*, and this chain binds to the *Fc fragment* of IgE with high *affinity*. The β chain is a *Type III transmembrane protein* with four membrane-spanning domains. The γ chains are identical to the γ chain of FcγRIII (see *Fcγ receptors*). FcεRI is found on *mast cells, basophil leucocytes, Langerhans cells* and stimulated *eosinophil leucocytes*. Binding to IgE has no biological effects until the IgE (and thus the receptor) is cross linked by binding to *antigen*. In mast cells this results in cellular degranulation, release of *vascular permeability factors*, of many *cytokines*, and synthesis of *leukotrienes*. In stimulated eosinophils it leads to release of cytoplasmic granules. (b) FcεRII. Low affinity IgE receptor. *CD23* q.v.

Fcγ receptors (IgG Fc receptors, FcγR) There are three distinct Fcγ receptors. All are active in opsonic phagocytosis of *IgG* coated particles (see *opsonization*), cytotoxicity and generation of a metabolic burst in phagocytic cells (see *phagocytosis*). The binding *affinity* of all three receptors in man is higher for IgG subclasses IgG1 and IgG3 than for IgG2 and IgG4 (see *immunoglobulin subclass*). In the mouse FcγRI and II bind IgG2a most strongly while FcγRIII binds IgG3, 2a and 2b. Mouse IgG1 is weakly bound. All these Fcγ receptors are also released from cells in soluble form.

(a) **FcγRI** (CD64). An Fc receptor constitutively expressed on *monocytes* and *macrophages* only, but which may be expressed on *neutrophil leucocytes* or *eosinophil leucocytes* following activation by *cytokines* such as **IFN-γ**. A *Type I transmembrane protein* of the *Ig superfamily*. Binds monomeric IgG with high affinity.

(b) **FcγRII** (CD32). Found constitutively on most leucocytes, e.g. monocytes, macrophages, neutrophil leucocytes, eosinophil leucocytes, *basophil leucocytes*, *B lymphocytes*, and *Langerhans cells*. A Type I transmembrane protein of the Ig superfamily. There are a number of variants (FcγRIIA, B and C to date). Binds polymeric or aggregated IgG.

(c) **FcγRIII** (CD16). Found constitutively in *GPI anchor*-linked form on neutrophil leucocytes (CD16b) and in Type I transmembrane form on *NK cells*, monocytes, macrophages and some T cells (CD16a). It is a member of the Ig superfamily and is non-covalently associated with a γ chain (similar to the γ chain of FcεRI, see *Fcε receptors*) and the ζ (zeta) *chain* that is also associated with *TCR*. It is present on eosinophil leucocytes following activation with IFN-γ. It is a low affinity receptor for polymerized IgG (*immune complexes*).

Fd fragment The portion of the *heavy chain* of an *immunoglobulin* molecule N-terminal to the site of papain hydrolysis (cf. *Fc fragment* and see Figure I2). It contains the *variable region* and part of the *constant region*.

ferritin labelling See *immunoferritin technique*.

first set rejection The *immunological rejection* of an organ or tissue that has been grafted onto a previously **unprimed** host. Cf. *second set rejection*.

FITC Fluorescein isothiocyanate. A reactive *fluorescein* derivative which combines with proteins in alkaline solution. Used for preparing *fluorescein labelled*

antibody, etc. for *immunofluorescence* q.v.

FK506® A macrolide antibiotic derived from the fungus *Streptomyces tsukubaensis* first isolated from the slopes of Mt Fujiyama. It has closely similar *immunosuppressive* actions to those of *cyclosporin A*, and blocks *T cell* activation and *cytokine* gene expression early in the G1 phase of growth by inhibiting *calcineurin* phosphatase. Binds to *FKBP* and its action is mediated by the drug–protein complex.

FKBP *FK506*®-binding protein. There are several related intracellular FKBPs. Once they bind FK506®, the drug–protein complex binds to *calcineurin* and inhibits its action in *T cells*, thus inducing *immunosuppression*. FKBPs and *cyclophilins* are known collectively as immunophilins.

flagellin Protein, forming major constituent of flagella of motile bacteria. Used as experimental *antigen*. The monomeric form is a *thymus dependent antigen* whereas polymerized flagellin is a *thymus independent antigen*, see also *TI-2 antigen*.

flow cytometry The measurement of the size and refractive index of individual cells in a fluid stream. These cells intersect a laser beam and reflected light is collected by a photomultiplier tube set at right angles to the fluid stream, hence 'side scatter' or '90° scatter'. Refracted light around the cell is proportional to size and is collected incident to the laser beam, hence 'forward scatter'. If the cells are incubated with a fluorescent protein, usually an *antibody* against a specific cell surface *antigen* this can be excited by the high energy laser light and the Stokes-shift emitted light is collected. Up to three distinct wavelengths can normally be detected, allowing cellular discrimination according to five parameters. The collected light from each cell is converted into electronic analogue data which is processed by computer and can be presented as coordinates on a dot plot or as a histogram on screen.

fluorescein A yellow dye with an intense green fluorescence. Reactive derivatives of it are used for labelling proteins for *immunofluorescence* tests. See *FITC, fluorochrome*.

fluorescein labelled antibody *Antibody* to which fluorescein has been covalently linked usually in the form of an isothiocyanate (see *FITC*) or isocyanate. Used in *immunofluorescence* tests.

fluorescence activated cell sorter (FACS) A flow cytometer (see *flow cytometry*) which can be programmed to collect a specified cell population from a mixture by charge deflection after they have been selected according to the desired characteristics of size and refractive index as well as by a fluorescent probe, most commonly a conjugated *antibody* to a cell surface antigen. Also widely used for determining the phenotype of cell populations, and the proportions of *CD4+* and *CD8+ T lymphocytes, B lymphocytes, monocytes, NK cells*, etc. using appropriate *monoclonal antibodies* and a *double labelling* technique when applicable.

fluorescent antibody technique *Immunofluorescence* (q.v.) technique in which *antibody* conjugated to a *fluorochrome* is used to locate *antigen* in tissue sections or cell preparations.

fluorochrome A substance which emits visible light of a characteristic wavelength when irradiated with a shorter wavelength. Fluorochromes are used as labels for other molecules since they can be observed in trace amounts. See *fluorescein, phycoerythrin, rhodamines*.

fluorography Technique used to detect radiolabelled molecules, especially proteins and nucleic acids, after separation by electrophoresis in gels and *immunoblotting, Southern blotting* or *northern blotting*. For high energy isotopes (^{125}I, ^{32}P) a plastic screen coated with a 'fluor', a substance that emits photons on exposure to radiation, is placed on the opposite side of a sheet of X-ray film to the gel or membrane. After exposure for a period of a few hours to several days the X-ray film is developed and blackening is observed in regions corresponding to the radiolabelled molecules. Commonly used for the detection of *antigens* by overlay with radiolabelled *antibody*, or of genes and mRNA after Southern and northern blotting. For low energy isotopes (^{3}H, ^{14}C, ^{35}S) the gel itself can be impregnated with the fluor and dried. More sensitive than *autoradiography*.

follicle Spherical accumulation of *lymphocytes* in *lymphoid tissues*. See *lymph node, spleen, primary follicle, secondary follicle, germinal centre*.

follicular dendritic cell (FDC) A cell with extensive dendritic processes found in the *B cell* areas of *lymphoid tissue*, i.e. in *primary follicles* and *germinal centres*. Follicular dendritic cells are not *bone marrow*-derived and are unrelated to the *dendritic cells* (q.v.) found in *T cell* areas and in other parts of the body (e.g. *Langerhans cells, veiled cells, interdigitating cells*). They are long-lived cells which can hold antigen in the form of *immune complexes* on their surfaces for long periods. During an *immune response*, they present *antigen* in these complexes to B cells. B cells with high *affinity* for the antigen survive and differentiate to *antibody*-secreting or *memory cells*. Other B cells die by *apoptosis*. Follicular dendritic cells have *Fc receptors* and *C3b receptors* but, unlike other dendritic cells, they do not process or present antigen in a way that allows *recognition* by T cells.

follicular hyperplasia Local or generalized enlargement of *lymph nodes* with increase in size and number of the *follicles* which typically contain active *germinal centres* (q.v.). This is a reactive change in the lymph nodes, usually following infection and is distinguishable from the *lymphomas*.

follicular mantle See *mantle zone*.

food allergy *Hypersensitivity* (often *type I hypersensitivity reaction*) to constituents of food. Ingestion of food containing *allergens* may be followed immediately by distress, buccal oedema, diarrhoea and vomiting or later by generalized manifestations such as *urticaria* or *eczema*. Many foods, especially fish, nuts or eggs, may cause such symptoms, children being particularly susceptible to eggs. Detected by skin tests using an extract containing the appropriate *antigen* (allergen) or RAST testing (*radioallergosorbent test*). Confirmation by exclusion diet is often required but only under the supervision of a dietician.

forbidden clone Hypothetical clone of *lymphocytes* with specificity for *auto-antigens* which, according to the *clonal selection theory*, have been suppressed in fetal life and which may regain activity in adult life and cause *auto-immune disease*.

formyl peptides Synthetic formyl peptides (type example: formyl-Met-Leu-Phe) are strong chemotactic factors (see *chemotaxis*) for *neutrophil leucocytes* and *mononuclear phagocytes*. These cells possess specific *rhodopsin super-family* receptors for them. May be analogues of chemotactic peptides released from pathogenic bacteria.

Forssman antigen A glycolipid *antigen* present on tissue cells of many species, e.g. horse, sheep, mouse, dog and cat, but absent in man, rabbit, rat, pig and cow.

framework region The sequence of amino acids in *immunoglobulin* and *TCR* variable regions surrounding the three *hypervariable regions*. The framework region is more conserved than the hypervariable regions and is responsible for the basic secondary and tertiary structure of the *variable region* domain

(see *homology region*). It is believed to contribute less than the hypervariable regions to the structure of the *antigen-binding site*.

freemartin The female of twin bovine calves where the other twin is male and the two placentae have become fused *in utero*. Thus the twins have exchanged cells before immunological maturity and are *chimeras* that do not reject grafts made from each other. In this situation the female calf is sterile due, amongst other things, to the influence of male hormones and can be recognized by physical examination.

Freund's adjuvant See *complete Freund's adjuvant* and *incomplete Freund's adjuvant*.

functional affinity The *affinity* of an *antibody* as determined by a technique that does not give a direct measurement of the free interaction between a single *epitope* or *hapten* and a single *antigen-binding site*, e.g. using the *ELISA* assay, in which the *antigen* is usually multi-valent and in the solid phase coated on plastic. The antibody–antigen interaction, therefore, includes a cooperative effect between the antigen binding sites and the result is a measure of antibody *avidity* rather than true affinity.

functional immunity See *protective immunity*.

fyn A *protein tyrosine kinase*, (member of the Src family) which associates with the *TCR/CD3* ζ (zeta) *chain* and is involved in antigen-induced *T cell* signalling.

G

G-CSF (granulocyte colony stimulating factor) A cytokine made chiefly by *mononuclear phagocytes*, e.g. following stimulation by *IFN-γ*, *TNF-α* or *lipopolysaccharide*, whose major action is on the *bone marrow* precursors of *neutrophil leucocytes*, in which it induces proliferation and differentiation to mature neutrophils. Thus its action is subsequent to, and more specific, than that of *GM-CSF*. Shares sequence homology with *IL-6*.

G-CSFR (granulocyte colony stimulating factor receptor) A *Type I transmembrane protein* with an *immunoglobulin* domain, a *cytokine* receptor domain and four fibronectin-like domains. Two forms have been identified differing in their cytoplasmic regions. Found on *neutrophil leucocytes* and their *bone marrow* precursors

G proteins (GTP-binding proteins) These regulate many cellular functions by changing conformation from an inactive GDP-bound form to an active GTP-bound form. There are two classes, the trimeric and the monomeric G proteins. Trimeric proteins consist of α, β and γ subunits and couple *receptors* to enzymes involved in generating second messengers. On binding of a *ligand* by the receptor, the α subunit of the G protein binds GTP and can then activate enzymes, e.g. adenylate cyclase which generates cyclic AMP, or phospholipase C which generates inositol phosphates and diacylglycerol thus mobilizing Ca^{2+} and activating *protein kinase C*. These events regulate many functions in immune cells. Trimeric G proteins are directly activated by receptors of the *rhodopsin superfamily*. Monomeric G proteins have many functions. One group, the Ras protein family, is involved in signal relay from protein tyrosine kinases and may regulate *lym-phocyte activation* and cell motility *inter alia*.

GALT See *gut associated lymphoid tissue*.

γ (gamma) **chain disease** A rare *paraproteinaemia* in man associated with *lymphoma* in which abnormal monoclonal γ chains (i.e. *heavy chains* of *IgG*) are found in the *plasma* and urine in the absence of *light chains*. The γ chains contain a deletion in which most of the *variable region* and all of the C_H1 region are absent although some of the N-terminal amino acids are still present. The *hinge region* is also sometimes missing.

γ globulin See *gamma globulin*.

γδ T cells Lineage of *T lymphocyte* possessing the γδ form of the T cell receptor (*TCR*). Appears early in ontogeny, during *thymus* development, and also accounts for about 5% of mature T lymphocytes in *peripheral lymphoid organs*. In many species, γδ T cells may be the predominant population of T lymphocyte at epithelial surfaces, such as the skin, intestine and genital tract. Some of these γδ T cells may be extrathymically derived. Most γδ T cells express neither *CD4* nor *CD8* molecules and their recognition specificities and functions are unknown. γδ T cells never express the αβ TCR and they constitute a separate lineage of T cells.

γ_m The membrane form of the γ chain (*heavy chain*) of *IgG*.

γ_s The secreted form of the γ chain (*heavy chain*) of *IgG*.

gamma (γ) **globulin** The *globulin* fraction of *serum* that on electrophoresis shows the lowest anodic mobility at neutral pH. Contains mainly *immunoglobulins*.

gel diffusion test *Precipitin test* in which *antigen* and *antibody* are placed in a gel of agar or similar substance and allowed to diffuse towards one another to form a precipitate. See *double diffusion test, reaction of identity, Ouchterlony test*.

gene knockout mouse A mouse in which a selected gene has been replaced by an inactive mutant and which therefore lacks the protein coded for by that gene. The mutant gene is introduced with a vector into embryonic *stem cells* in culture which are then implanted *in vivo* and allowed to undergo fetal development. The resulting offspring which are found to be homozygous for the gene defect are bred. Gene knockout mice are used in immunology and elsewhere for studies of the effects of lack of function of specified proteins. They are referred to by prefixing with the missing product, e.g. 'perforin-knockout mice'. See also *transgenic mouse*.

germ free Reared in the complete absence of bacteria and larger organisms. Freedom from all viruses is more difficult to achieve. Cf. *gnotobiotic, axenic*.

germinal centre A spherical aggregation of *B lymphocytes* which develops within the *primary follicles* of *lymphoid tissues* in response to stimulation by *thymus dependent antigens* (see Figures L1 and S1). Following antigen *recognition* in the *T cell* area, B cells migrate to the primary follicles where they proliferate massively to form a germinal centre, displacing the small recirculating B cells into the *mantle zone* (follicular mantle). After several days, the centre characteristically contains a dark zone with few *follicular dendritic cells* (FDC) but rich in *centroblasts*, and a light zone containing a network of antigen-bearing FDC together with *centrocytes* which make contact with antigen on the FDC (see Figure G1). The germinal centre is the site of *isotype switching* and *affinity maturation* of B cells. Those cells with high *affinity* for *antigen* are positively selected (see *positive selection*) and survive. The rest die by *apoptosis* and are removed by *tingible body macrophages*.

The B cells in germinal centres are oligoclonal suggesting response to a single antigen. Following selection cells may leave the germinal centre as *plasmablasts* which migrate to the *medullary cords* or the *bone marrow*, or as B *memory cells* many of which are found in the *marginal zone*. Note that there are enough T cells in germinal centres to allow interactions between T and B cells (e.g. between *CD40L* and *CD40*).

germinal follicle Synonym for *germinal centre*.

gld A mutation of the gene for the *Fas* ligand (see *TNF family*) which prevents it from binding to Fas and hence blocks *apoptosis*, causing uncontrolled proliferation of *T cells* in mice homozygous for this mutation. Such mice develop an *autoimmune disease* resembling **SLE** (systemic lupus erythematosus), cf. *MRL-lpr/lpr mice* and *lpr^{cg}*. Gld stands for 'generalized lymphoproliferative disease'.

globulin Any *serum* protein whose anodic mobility on electrophoresis is less than that of albumin. Includes α, β and γ globulins; the latter fraction includes the *immunoglobulins*. Also commonly used to define those serum proteins which are precipitated by high concentrations of salts such as ammonium or sodium sulphate. Euglobulins are proteins (including *IgM* but not the other classes of immunoglobulins) which are precipitated in distilled water or solutions of low ionic strength. These definitions are less precise than the electrophoretic definition. Cf. *albumin*.

glomerulonephritis A term applied, with various qualifying prefixes, to a group of kidney diseases, in which the major lesion is in the glomeruli and is presumed to be immunologically mediated. This is supported by work carried out in experimental animals in which the glomerular capillaries are specially susceptible to deposition of circulating soluble *immune complexes*, with consequent injury (as in *serum sickness*). Glomerulonephritis has also been produced experimentally by injection of

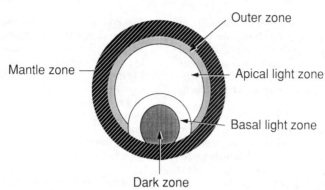

Figure G1. Germinal centre.

antibody to capillary basement membrane, and by *immunization* with basement membrane. See also *streptococcal nephritis*.

GlyCAM-1 (glycosylation-dependent cell adhesion molecule-1) A heavily glycosylated transmembrane molecule found selectively on **high endothelial venules** of peripheral *lymph nodes*. It binds to L-selectin (see *selectins*) on *lymphocytes*, and binding requires that the GlyCAM-1 molecule be sialylated. Probably important for the homing of recirculating lymphocytes (see *lymphocyte recirculation*) into peripheral *lymphoid tissues*.

Gm allotype (Gm group) An allotypic *epitope* on the *heavy chain* (γ chain) of human *IgG*. First discovered by observation of varying reactions of *rheumatoid factor* with IgG from different donors. 25 Gm *allotypes* are known, viz. Gm (1), Gm(2), etc. Many Gm allotypes have been shown to be confined to a particular IgG subclass (see *immunoglobulin subclass*) but some are shared between different subclasses. Many of the Gm allotypes have been correlated with single or multiple amino acid substitutions at various positions in the *constant region* of the heavy chain. They can occur in any of the three constant region domains.

GM-CSF (granulocyte–macrophage colony stimulating factor) A *cytokine* made by *lymphocytes*, *macrophages* and other cell types which is necessary for differentiation of myeloid (see *myeloid cell series*) lineage-specific *bone marrow* stem cells to form *neutrophil leucocytes*, *mononuclear phagocytes* and *eosinophil leucocytes*. The final pathway taken by these precursors is determined by other cytokines, e.g. *G-CSF, M-CSF*. Also required for growth and differentiation of *dendritic cell* precursors. It also has peripheral actions and will activate and enhance the survival of mature neutrophils and eosinophils. It acts as a neutrophil primer (see *priming*[2]) and enhances phagocytic activity (see *phagocytosis*) and *ADCC* activity in mature myeloid cells.

GM-CSFR (granulocyte–macrophage colony stimulating factor receptor; CDw116) A *Type I transmembrane protein* (heterodimeric) of the *cytokine receptor superfamily* found on *monocytes*, *macrophages*, *neutrophil leucocytes*, *eosinophil leucocytes* and *bone marrow* myeloid precursors (see *myeloid cell series*). Has a unique α chain and a β chain common to itself, *IL-3* and *IL-5*.

gnotobiotic Descriptive of an environment in which all of the living organisms present are known, e.g. both a *germ free* mouse, and a mouse contaminated with a single known organism, may be described as gnotobiotic.

Goodpasture's syndrome Haemoptysis (coughing up blood) associated with proliferative *glomerulonephritis*. The glomerular basement membrane is thickened and *IgG* and, to a lesser extent, *complement* are deposited in a linear fashion along the basement membrane.

GPI anchor (glycosyl-phosphatidyl-inositol) A structure through which membrane proteins lacking a trans-membrane domain are integrated into the cell membrane. The extracellular protein is covalently linked to a short sugar sequence which terminates in phosphatidylinositol, the fatty acid tails of which are incorporated into the lipid bilayer. Thus GPI-linked membrane proteins have no cytoplasmic tail. Among important proteins linked in this way are the mouse *T cell* marker, *Thy-1*, the FcγRIII (in *neutrophil leucocytes*, see *Fcγ receptors*), *LFA-3* and *CD14*. See Figure T3.

graft rejection Destruction of tissue grafted into a genetically dissimilar recipient due to a specific *immunological reaction* against it by the recipient.

graft-versus-host disease The clinical disease resulting from the *graft-versus-host reaction* which occurs in human recipients of *allogeneic bone marrow* transplants. It is associated with damage to the skin, intestine and liver and causes profound *immunosuppression*.

graft-versus-host reaction Reaction of a graft containing immunologically competent *T lymphocytes*, against the tissues of a genetically non-identical recipient. The recipient must be unable to reject the graft either because of its immaturity (newborn animals, see *runt disease*), or its genetic constitution, or because it has been subjected to whole body irradiation or *immunosuppression*.

granulocyte One of a group of *bone marrow*-derived cells found in blood and tissues and characterized by the presence of numerous cytoplasmic granules. Three types of granulocyte can be differentiated by the morphology and staining properties of these granules (which give them their name); thus neutrophil, eosinophil and basophil granulocytes (see under their synonyms *neutrophil leucocyte, eosinophil leucocyte* and *basophil leucocyte*). The functions of these three types are quite different.

granuloma The term is most frequently used to refer to a localized collection of *macrophages* and *lymphocytes* characteristic of chronic inflammatory lesions in which a *delayed-type hypersensitivity* (DTH) reaction is taking place, as in tuberculosis and other chronic infections or in lesions of *autoimmunity*. Granulomata that form in response to foreign bodies and chronic infections, often show special features. Thus foreign body granulomata have a very high proportion of giant cells, tuberculous granulomata contain *epithelioid cells* and Langhans giant cells and syphilitic granulomata are heavily infiltrated by lymphocytes and *plasma cells*. See also *adjuvant granuloma*.

granzyme Granzymes are a family of serine proteases found in the granules of cytolytic *lymphocytes (cytotoxic T lymphocytes, NK cells)* and which are believed to play a part in lymphocyte-mediated cytotoxicity. They share some sequence homology with *serprocidins* (q.v.) in *neutrophil leucocytes* and *macrophages*.

GRO See Table C2.

gut associated lymphoid tissue (GALT) *Lymphoid tissue* closely associated with the gut, e.g. *tonsils, Peyer's patches* and appendix in man, sacculus rotundus in the rabbit, *bursa of Fabricius* in the chicken, etc.

GVH See *graft-versus-host reaction*.

H

H chain See *heavy chain*.

H-2 histocompatibility system The *major histocompatibility system* in the mouse, H-2 genes determine the major histocompatibility antigens on somatic cell surfaces and also the level of *immune response* of the animal (*Ir genes*). The antigens borne by a given strain of mouse, i.e. its H-2 type, are controlled by the arrangement of alleles within this locus and grafts between different H-2 types suffer *immunological rejection* (see **H-2D, H-2I, H-2K** and Figure H1. Cf. also *HLA histocompatibility system*).

H-2 restriction *MHC restriction* (q.v.) applied to the mouse *H-2 histocompatibility system*.

H-2D A genetic locus in the H-2 major histocompatibility complex of the mouse (see *H-2 histocompatibility system* and Figure H1). H-2D products are *class I MHC antigens*. There are numerous alleles at *H-2D*, e.g. *H-2D^b* (abbreviated:

D^b), *H-2D^q* (*D^q*), etc. Designations of loci and alleles are set in italic, designations of their products in roman print, (e.g. the *H-2D^b* allele encodes the H-2D^b antigen). See also **H-2K**.

H-2I region In the murine *major histocompatibility complex* (MHC) the I region includes many of the genes coding for *class II MHC antigens*. Five separate genes are recognized (see *H-2 histocompatibility system* and Figure H1), $A\alpha$, $A\beta$, $E\alpha$, $E\beta$, and $E\beta2$; the equivalents in man are the HLA, DP, DQ and DR regions. The involvement of the products of this region in many aspects of the *immunological response* gave it the general name 'I = immune' region. See also *Ir gene*.

H-2K A genetic locus in the H-2 major histocompatibility complex of mouse (see *H-2 histocompatibility system* and Figure H1). H-2K products are *class I antigens*. There are numerous alleles at *H-2K*, e.g. *H-2K^b* (abbreviated: K^b), *H-2K^q*

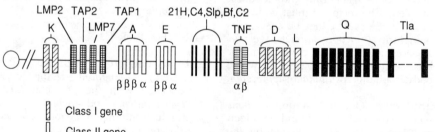

Figure H1. Legend:
- Class I gene
- Class II gene
- Class III gene
- Non-classical class I gene (less polymorphic than classical class I genes) The number of Tla genes varies between mouse strains.
- TAP and proteasome (LMP) genes
- O Centromere

Figure H1. H-2 histocompatibility system. Map of the mouse H-2 histocompatibility gene locus. Genes are shown as boxes, non-coding regions as a horizontal straight line. Only the important genes are shown. Not to scale.

(K^q) etc. See also **H-2D** for the conventions used in these designations.

H-2L Class I murine histocompatibility antigen, coded for by locus closely linked to **H-2D** (see **H-2 histocompatibility system** and Figure H1). Detectable on **spleen** cells, and can be recognized as target determinant for **graft rejection** or in cytotoxic killing assay (see **cytotoxicity tests**). Serological cross reactivity occurs with **H-2D** and **H-2K** products.

haemagglutination *Agglutination* of erythrocytes (red blood cells).

haemagglutination test *Agglutination* test in which *antibody* reacts with *antigen* on the surface of erythrocytes. See also *passive agglutination test* and *tanned red cell test*.

haemagglutinin (1) *Agglutinin¹* of red blood cells. (2) Non-*antibody* substance, e.g. a *lectin* or a surface component of a virus particle that has the ability to agglutinate erythrocytes.

haemocyanin The oxygen-carrying blood pigment of invertebrates; often used as an experimental *antigen* in mammals.

haemocyte Generic term used in invertebrate biology for *leucocytes*, both circulating and sessile. Associated with the mechanisms of internal defence such as *phagocytosis* and *encapsulation* in animals such as arthropods and molluscs, which have a large 'open' blood system (haemocoele). See also *coelomocyte*.

haemocytoblast Synonym for *stem cell* in *bone marrow* and other haemopoietic tissues.

haemolysin (1) *Antibody* capable of lysing erythrocytes in presence of *complement*. (2) Term also used of other substances, e.g. bacterial toxins, which cause haemolysis.

haemolysis Lysis (bursting of cell membrane and cell death) of erythrocytes.

haemolytic anaemia Anaemia due to an abnormal increase in the rate of destruction of circulating erythrocytes. Can result from metabolic abnormalities of the erythrocytes, from the development of *antibodies* to the erythrocytes, or from abnormalities of the *mononuclear phagocyte* system. Haemolytic anaemia due to isoantibodies (i.e. antibodies against *isoantigen*) occurs in *erythroblastosis fetalis* and can also result from mismatched blood or plasma transfusion. Autoimmune haemolytic anaemia results from the development of *autoantibody* to erythrocytes; it may develop as a primary disease, or as a complication of various conditions, including lymphoid neoplasms, primary atypical pneumonia, etc. The destruction of erythrocytes in haemolytic anaemia may be due to intravascular *haemolysis* or to *phagocytosis* by mononuclear phagocytes in the liver and spleen. In bacterial (and possibly some protozoal) infections, antigen from the organism may coat the host's erythrocytes so that the subsequent antibody response destroys them as well as the bacteria.

haemolytic disease of the newborn *Haemolytic anaemia* in the fetus or newborn resulting from an access of maternal anti red cell *antibody*. In man, occurs due to antibody, (usually Rhesus antibody; see **Rhesus blood group system**) crossing the placenta, see *erythroblastosis fetalis*. In the horse and the pig, follows the neonatal ingestion of *colostrum*, as, in these species, antibody does not cross the placenta. In man giving *anti-D* to the mother soon after parturition prevents haemolytic disease in a subsequent pregnancy.

haemolytic plaque assay See *plaque-forming cell assay*.

haemolytic system The mixture of sheep erythrocytes and specific *antibody* to them that is used as an indicator of the presence or absence of *complement* in the second stage of a *complement fixation test* q.v.

haemopoietic growth factors See *GM-CSF, M-CSF* and *IL-3*.

haemopoietin receptor family See *cytokine receptor superfamily*.

haplotype (haploid genotype) A cluster of *MHC genes* inherited from one parent which, because of their close linkage on the same chromosome, are normally inherited together. Each somatic cell has two haplotypes, one paternally derived and the other maternally derived. Some haplotypes show strong *linkage disequilibrium* between alleles of different loci.

hapten Substance that can combine with *antibody*, but cannot initiate an *immune response* unless it is bound to a *carrier* before introduction into the body. Most haptens are small molecules (MW <1 kD). Haptenic groups can be conjugated to carriers *in vitro* and require the carrier molecule to become *immunogenic in vivo*.

hapten inhibition test Any *inhibition test* technique by means of which an *epitope* is characterized serologically or its molecular configuration elucidated by using *haptens* of known structure to block the combining site of an *antibody* directed against it, e.g. oligosaccharides may be used in such a test to discover the sugar sequences that determine specificity in polysaccharide *antigens*.

haptotaxis This term was originally introduced to define locomotion of cells on a surface bearing a gradient of adhesiveness. It is now generally used to define *chemotaxis* along a gradient in which the attractant molecules are surface-bound rather than in free solution.

Hashimoto's thyroiditis A disease of the human thyroid characterized by chronic inflammatory change, including infiltration with *lymphocytes, plasma cells* and *macrophages*, and sometimes formation of *germinal centres*. The gland is enlarged and firm. The acinar epithelium may be increased, but is progressively destroyed and thyroid function is commonly depressed. It is considered to be an *autoimmune disease*, and *autoantibodies* against thyroid antigens (thyroglobulin, acinar cell microsomal antigen, thyroid colloid) are present in the *serum* in most cases. Related to non-progressive focal chronic thyroiditis, and to primary hypothyroidism which is probably an atrophic variant.

Hassall's corpuscles Keratinized epithelial whorls or islands of cells found in the medulla of the *thymus*. These may be end-stage *thymic epithelial cells* and are associated with *macrophages* and apoptotic (see *apoptosis*) *lymphocytes*. Thus the Hassall's corpuscle may be a site of removal of dead cells.

HAT selection HAT is an abbreviation for hypoxanthine, aminopterin and thymidine. The HAT selection technique is used to select for cells which have fused with a cell line, e.g. in the production of *monoclonal antibody*-secreting *hybridomas* or *T cell* hybridomas. The fusion partner is a *plasmacytoma* or T *lymphoma* cell line deficient in the enzyme hypoxanthine guanine phosphoribosyl transferase (HGPRT), necessary for purine synthesis, and thus unable to grow in medium containing HAT. After fusion, the fused normal *plasma cell* or *lymphocyte* provides the HGPRT thus enabling the hybrid cell to grow in the presence of HAT.

hay fever Acute nasal catarrh and conjunctivitis in *atopic* subjects caused by the inhalation of antigenic substances such as pollens (*allergens* q.v.) that are innocuous in normal persons. Due to *immediate hypersensitivity* (*type I hypersensitivity reaction*) following the reaction of cell-fixed *IgE* with the causative allergen. Often seasonal depending on concentration of the relevant antigen in air.

HD$_{50}$ More usually known as *CH$_{50}$* (q.v.)

heat aggregated protein antigen Protein antigen whose antigenicity has been modified by mild heating, e.g. to 63°C. This causes some denaturation, makes the protein less soluble and reveals new *epitopes*. *Rheumatoid factor* (q.v.) is an *autoantibody* which reacts *in vitro* with heat-aggregated *gamma globulin* more strongly than with native gamma globulin.

heat inactivation Destruction of biological activity by heating. Especially, in immunology, the destruction of *complement* activity by heating serum to 56°C for 20 minutes. This inactivates the heat-labile factors *C1*, *C2* and *Factor B*.

heat shock proteins (HSP) Ubiquitous intracellular proteins in all species, whose level increases when the organism is stressed. They were first identified following heat stress. They are highly conserved, nevertheless there is enough variation for heat shock proteins made by pathogenic bacteria and protozoa to be strong *antigens* in mammals (e.g. HSP65 of *Mycobacterium tuberculosis* is the major antigen of the bacterium). They are involved in repair and re-folding of denatured proteins and they also assist in the folding and assembly of normal proteins, hence classified as 'chaperonins'. In immune cells they assist in the assembly of *immunoglobulin* molecules and are believed to play an important role in *antigen processing* inasmuch as they assist the intracellular assembly of *major histocompatibility complex* (MHC) molecules.

heavy chain A polypeptide chain present in all *immunoglobulin* molecules. MW approx. 50 kD in human *IgG*, 65 kD in *IgM*. Each heavy chain is normally linked by disulphide bonds to a *light chain* and to another identical heavy chain (see Figure I2). The heavy chain consists of a *variable region* (V_H) and a *constant region* composed of three or four domains (C_H1–C_H4) depending on *immunoglobulin class*. The amino acid sequence of the heavy chain constant region determines the class and *immunoglobulin subclass*, and the corresponding heavy chain is called the α chain, δ chain, ε chain, γ chain, or μ chain.

heavy chain class The group into which a *heavy chain* is placed by virtue of features of its primary or *antigenic* structure, common to all individuals of the same species, which distinguish it from heavy chains of other classes. These structural differences are found in the *constant region*. The heavy chain classes are α, δ, ε, γ and μ. See also *immunoglobulin class* and *isotype*.

heavy chain disease See α *chain disease*, γ *chain disease*.

helper T lymphocyte (T_H lymphocyte, helper cell) A thymus-derived lymphocyte (usually *CD4+*, *class II MHC antigen*-restricted, see *MHC restriction*) whose presence (help) is required for the production of normal levels of *antibody* by *B lymphocytes* and also for the normal development of cell-mediated immunity. This help requires the production of *cytokines* such as *IL-4*, *IL-5* and *IL-6* or *IL-2* and *IFN-γ*. See T_H1 *cells* and T_H2 *cells*.

hemagglutination, etc. American spelling of haemagglutination, etc.

herd immunity A concept embracing a variety of factors that make a large natural group of persons or animals (the herd) insusceptible to infection. It may, therefore, have nothing to do with *specific immunity*. Thus, herd immunity may be brought about by providing pure water or good drainage and, e.g. epidemics of plague no longer occur because in modern societies the man–flea–rat contact has been broken. Specific immunity may, however, play a part in herd immunity, e.g. when a sufficiently large percentage of the herd is *immune[1]*, epidemics cannot spread.

hereditary angio-oedema Disease transmitted as Mendelian dominant, characterized by recurrent, acute, circumscribed transient oedema of skin and mucosae. May threaten life in its laryngeal form. Two forms exist: Type I is associated with low levels of *C1 inhibitor* production. Type II is associated with normal levels of an *inactive* C1 inhibitor molecule. Low serum levels of *C2* and *C4* are found, especially during attacks. Note that C1 inhibitor is also an inhibitor of the *kinin* system which may be responsible for the symptoms.

heteroclitic antibody *Antibody* produced in response to *immunization* with one *antigen* that has higher *affinity* for another antigen that was not present during the immunization. The second antigen may have a molecular structure related to that used for immunization.

heterogeneic See *xenogeneic* (preferred term).

heterograft See *xenograft* (preferred term) and *transplantation terminology*.

heterologous Derived from a different species.

heterologous carrier vaccine *Vaccine* which is attached to and delivered on another macromolecule (the carrier) in order to enhance its *immunogenicity*. The carriers are either large *immunogenic* protein molecules or live attenuated viruses or bacteria (see *attenuated vaccine*). The target *antigen* of the vaccine is attached covalently on to the protein carrier, or the gene for it is cloned directly into an expression plasmid which is then transfected into the live *heterologous* carrier. The carrier primes *helper T lymphocytes* which enhance *humoral immunity* or *cell-mediated immunity* against the target antigen.

heterologous vaccine Any *vaccine* which protects against pathogens not present in the vaccine. Contains microorganisms which share *cross reacting antigens* with the pathogen in question. Examples include the use of *vaccinia* in *smallpox vaccination*; of measles vaccine in canine distemper; of Shope fibroma virus against myxomatosis in rabbits.

heterospecific (heterologous) Derived from or having specificity for a different species.

heterotopic graft Organ or tissue grafted or transferred to an anatomical site where that organ or tissue is not normally found. Cf. *orthotopic graft*.

HEV See *high endothelial venule*.

HGG Human *gamma globulin*.

hidden determinant *Epitope* which is so positioned on a molecule or cell that it is not accessible for recognition by *lymphocytes* or *antibody* and is neither capable of binding specifically to them, nor of stimulating an *immune response*, unless some stereochemical change causes the hidden determinant to be revealed.

high dose tolerance Acquired tolerance following the administration of very large single (polysaccharide) or repeated (protein) doses of *antigen* to *immunologically competent* animals. Cf. *low dose tolerance*.

high endothelial venule (HEV) Specialized venules found in the *thymus dependent area* of the *lymph node* (see Figure L1). Characterized by prominent, cuboidal, high endothelial lining cells. Recirculation of lymphocytes from blood to lymph takes place through the walls of these vessels. High endothelial cells in lymphoid tissue at different sites (lymph nodes, *Peyer's patches*, etc.) carry specific adhesion molecules (*addressins*) which are recognized by *homing receptors* on lymphocytes, thus allowing different populations of lymphocytes to home in to specific lymphoid tissues.

high responder Term referring to *inbred strains* of mice which give strong *immune responses* to specified *antigens* (compared to other strains). Related to presence of *Ir genes* determining the response in question. Some Ir genes have been mapped to the *class II MHC antigen* locus and are believed to determine differences in *antigen presentation* by class II molecules. Other Ir genes map to the *immunoglobulin* loci and are probably related to differences in inherited *V exons*, *D exons* or *J exons*.

hinge region A flexible, proline-rich region of the *heavy chain* of the *immunoglobulin* molecule between the *Fab fragment* and the *Fc fragment* which acts as a hinge around which the Fab fragments can rotate. The angle between the Fab subunits may vary between 0° and 180°. The hinge region is adjacent to the sites of papain and pepsin hydrolysis (see Figure I2).

histamine A *vascular permeability factor*, vasodilator and smooth muscle constrictor, widely distributed in biological tissues and found in high concentration in *mast cells*. Histamine and histamine-like substances are released when cell-bound *IgE* reacts with *antigen*. They cause the classical vascular lesions (*weal and flare response*) of *immediate hypersensitivity*. *Anaphylatoxins* also mediate release of histamine.

histiocyte A pathologist's term for a macrophage found within the tissues, in contrast to those found in the blood (*monocytes*) or serous cavities, etc. Some histiocytes appear to remain at the same site for long periods of time, e.g. those that retain dye particles in the skin after tattooing. They have a strong affinity for silver and other heavy metal stains.

histocompatibility antigen Genetically determined *isoantigen* carried on the surface of nucleated cells of many tissues (and easily detected on blood *leucocytes*). Coded for by *MHC genes* (HLA, H-2) q.v. *Class I MHC antigens* and *class II MHC antigens* are of major importance in the *recognition* of and response to *antigens* by *T cells*, since the T cell receptor (*TCR*) recognizes antigenic peptides non-covalently bound in a cleft in these molecules. Also when tissue is grafted on to another individual of the same species whose tissues do not carry that antigen, it may incite an *immune response* which leads to *graft rejection*. The most closely studied histocompatibility antigens are those of the *H-2 histocompatibility system* in mice and of the *HLA histocompatibility system* in man.

histocompatibility gene Gene coding for a *histocompatibility antigen* q.v. See also *HLA histocompatibility system*, *H-2 histocompatibility system*.

histocompatibility locus Genetic locus on chromosome at which the histocompatibility genes which determine formation of histocompatibility antigens are situated. See *HLA* and *H-2 histocompatibility systems*.

histocompatibility testing The identification of *class I MHC antigens* and *class II MHC antigens* of the *HLA histocompatibility system* of man expressed on the cells of an individual. Used mainly to determine the compatibility of donor and recipient for transplantation of solid organs, of *bone marrow*, or for *platelet* transfusion, or for the assessment of disease associations. The commonest tests are serological, using panels of *antisera* against known HLA *antigens* to screen the *lymphocytes* of donor and recipient for their presence. A *cytotoxicity test* has been extensively used but this technique is now being replaced by *restriction fragment length polymorphism analysis* (RFLP) and the *polymerase chain reaction* (PCR). The *mixed leucocyte reaction, helper T lymphocyte* precursor (HTLp) and *cytotoxic T lymphocyte* precursor (CTLp) tests may also be used. HLA *antibody* identification and *cross matching* are also undertaken.

HIV (human immunodeficiency virus) A retrovirus belonging to the lentivirus family. HIV binds to the *CD4* molecule on *helper T lymphocytes* and also on *monocytes*. Binding allows entry of the virus into the CD4+ cell and may eventually cause destruction of that cell and thus a progressive reduction in CD4+ cell numbers. Lack of CD4+ cells leads to the symptoms of *AIDS*. There are two closely related viruses, HIV-1 and HIV-2, and probably others. HIV-1 is the common form in Europe and the USA, HIV-2 is common in West Africa.

HLA class I locus There are three well-defined loci for *class I MHC antigens* in man, viz. HLA-A, -B, and -C. Their protein products are found on all nucleated cells and present endogenous *antigenic* peptides to *CD8+ T lymphocytes* (see *antigen presentation*). In addition, HLA-E, -F, and -G are known to code for functional molecules. HLA-H and -J are pseudogenes. Over 96 specificities can be defined within the class I region by serological techniques. Note that the names of HLA genes are not italicized. See also *histocompatibility locus, MHC genes*.

HLA class II locus The HLA class II genes include DP, DQ and DR. Their protein products are expressed on *antigen-presenting cells* and inducible on other cells. They present exogenous *antigenic* peptides to *CD4+ T lymphocytes* (see *antigen presentation*). DQ and DR can be identified serologically although PCR (*polymerase chain* *reaction*) is increasingly being used. DP and DW, once only defined using the *mixed leucocyte reaction*, are also now identified using molecular probes. Over 76 specificities can be defined within the class II region. Note that the names of HLA genes are not italicized.

HLA histocompatibility system The *major histocompatibility complex* system of man, containing many genes which control the presence of cell surface *isoantigens*, as well as the capacity to mount immune responses (*Ir genes*). They are found on the short arm of chromosome 6 and are divided into three main groups: class I, class II and class III. Class I HLA antigens are encoded by the HLA-A, -B and -C genes, and are important in presentation of endogenous (e.g. viral) peptides to *CD8+ T lymphocytes* (see *antigen presentation*). The class II region includes HLA-DP, -DQ and -DR, which control presentation of exogenous antigens by specialized *antigen-presenting cells* (see also *class II MHC antigen*). HLA class I and class II antigens are important in tissue and organ transplantation since incompatibility of these antigens between donor and recipient may contribute to graft rejection. The A, B, C transporter genes *TAP1* and TAP2, and the DR transporter genes, DMA and DMB are also in this region. The class III region includes the *complement* genes *C2, C4* and Bf as well as Hsp70, *TNF*, LTB and CYP21. See Figure H2 for the arrangement of the more immunologically important genes. Many other genes are also present in this region. Note: the names of HLA system genes are not printed in italic as is the custom for other genes. Where, above, genes are marked as cross references this is to the product, not to the gene itself.

HML-1 (human mucosal antigen-1) An *integrin superfamily* protein found on *intraepithelial lymphocytes* composed of a β_7 integrin chain linked to a unique α chain (α_E; CD103).

Hodgkin's disease A *lymphoma*, characterized by the replacement of normal *lymphoid tissue* by neoplastic cells of which the typical example is the Reed–Sternberg giant cell, which is multinucleate, polyploid and phenotypically *class II MHC antigen+, CD15+, CD25+* and CD30+. The Reed–Sternberg cell has rearranged *V genes* for *immunoglobulin* suggesting that it originates from the *B lymphocyte* lineage. *Macrophages, neutrophil leucocytes, lymphocytes* and *eosinophil leucocytes* are also present and probably represent an inflammatory reaction against the neoplasm. There is enlargement of *lymph nodes* and *spleen* and infiltration of other tissues also occurs.

holoxenic Conventionally reared animals. Cf. *axenic, gnotobiotic*.

homing receptor The *receptor* or receptors on *leucocytes* that specifically recognize *addressins*, i.e. adhesion molecules on vascular endothelial cells; thus allowing specific entry of a leucocyte into a particular tissue. Term used especially in the context of *lymphocyte recirculation*.

homograft An outmoded term for any graft made from one individual to another of the same species. Included *allogeneic* grafts (*allografts*), and *syngeneic* grafts. The latter terms are more informative and used by transplantation immunologists. See also *transplantation terminology*.

homology region (immunoglobulin domain) A linear region of the *heavy chain* or *light chain* of the *immunoglobulin* molecule of approximately 105–115 amino acid residues which has a similar sequence to other regions of similar size. Each homology region contains one or more intrachain disulphide bonds and is folded to form a globular *domain* (q.v.) of similar shape. The homology regions are encoded by *exons* separated from each other by *introns* in germline DNA. Immunoglobulins probably evolved from a single gene, of the size of a homology region exon, by gene duplication. The homology regions of the light chains are designated V_L and C_L; those of the heavy chains V_H, C_H1, C_H2, etc. Similar regions characterize the many other proteins grouped within the *Ig superfamily*.

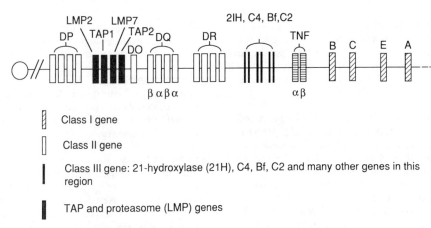

Figure H2. HLA histocompatibility system. Map of the human HLA histocompatibility gene locus. Genes are shown as boxes, non-coding regions as a horizontal straight line. Only the important genes are shown. Not to scale.

horror autotoxicus Concept introduced by Paul Ehrlich in 1901 affirming the existence of a mechanism whereby *autoantigens*, tissues and cells, potentially antigenic (see *antigen*) to other animals, do not cause a response of *autoimmunity* q.v.

house dust allergy Respiratory *hypersensitivity* reaction, e.g. *allergic rhinitis*, *asthma*, in *atopic* persons on inhalation of house dust. Chiefly of *immediate hypersensitivity* type (*type I hypersensitivity reaction*). Major *allergens* are proteases in the faecal pellets of the house dust mite *Dermatophagoides pteronyssinus* q.v.

HSA Human serum *albumin*. Frequently employed as an *antigen* in investigations with experimental animals. Immunologists also use this as an acronym for 'heat stable antigen', a *GPI-anchored* protein similar to CD24 and CDw52.

human immunodeficiency virus See *HIV*.

human umbilical vein endothelial cells (HUVEC) Endothelial cells prepared from the human umbilical vein are in frequent use as a model for studies of *leucocyte* adhesion (see *addressin*) to vascular endothelium.

humanized antibodies *Antibodies*, e.g. from rodents, that have been genetically engineered to make them more acceptable for use in man. (a) Chimeric (see *chimera*) *monoclonal antibodies* are constructed by grafting the *variable regions* of a rodent antibody on to the *constant regions* of a human antibody, thus reducing the *immunogenicity* of the rodent antibody for man and allowing selection of *immunoglobulin subclass* if any subclass-specific function is required. (b) The genes for the *hypervariable regions* (*complementarity determining regions*) of a rodent antibody can be grafted on to those for a human antibody. In this case only the *antigen-binding site* is foreign.

humoral antibody *Antibodies* present in the 'humours', i.e. *plasma*, *lymph* and tissue fluids of the body, and responsible for *humoral immunity*.

humoral immunity *Specific immunity* mediated by *antibodies*, and thus ultimately by *B lymphocytes*.

HUVEC See *human umbilical vein endothelial cells*.

hybrid antibodies *Immunoglobulin* molecules in which *antigen-binding sites* are of different specificities. Produced artificially by dissociating two *antibodies* of different specificities and then recombining them. Mixed immunoglobulin molecules are also produced by *hybridomas* resulting from the fusion of two immunoglobulin-producing cells. Not found naturally.

hybridoma (1) *B cell* hybridoma. A cell line obtained by the fusion of a *plasmacytoma* cell with a normal *plasma cell*. The latter is normally derived from an immunized animal. The resulting cell line continues to secrete the *antibody* produced by the plasma cell and has the immortality of the plasmacytoma cell. Since the hybridoma is a clone, the antibody produced is monoclonal, i.e. of unique sequence and specificity. Non-*immunoglobulin*-producing plasmacytoma cell lines are normally used as fusion partners since otherwise mixed products are obtained. Mouse, rat and human hybridomas have been successfully produced but hybridomas of mixed species tend to be unstable. See also *monoclonal antibody*. (2) *T cell* hybridoma. A cell line obtained by the fusion of a T *lymphoma* cell with a normal T lymphocyte.

5-hydroxytryptamine (5HT) See *serotonin*.

hyper-IgE syndrome A syndrome of recurrent, cold staphylococcal abscesses and other infections with persistent eczema, high serum *IgE* levels and a defect of *chemotaxis* of *neutrophil leucocytes*.

hypergammaglobulinaemia Raised *serum gamma globulin* level. Diffuse (i.e. not restricted to a single *immunoglobulin class*) increase in serum gamma globulin is associated with any condition where continued antigenic stimulation (see *antigen*) causes production of large amounts of *antibody*, e.g. chronic infection, *autoimmune diseases* and, irregularly, various chronic diseases of unknown causation. In *paraproteinaemias* a sharp, high electrophoretic spike of *immunoglobulin*, which is *monoclonal* in origin, is seen.

hyperimmune state A state, following repeated exposure to a single *antigen*, in which very large quantities of specific *antibody*, or very high levels of *cell-mediated immunity*, are present.

hyperimmunization Any method of *immunization[1]* designed to stimulate the production of very large quantities of *antibody* or very high levels of *cell-mediated immunity*.

hypersensitivity State of the previously immunized (see *immunization[1]*) body in which tissue damage results from the *immunological reaction* to a further dose of *antigen*. Hypersensitivity may be *antibody* mediated as in *immediate hypersensitivity* or in the *Arthus reaction* (see also *type I, II* and *III hypersensitivity reactions*) or it may be a reaction of *cell-mediated immunity* as in *delayed-type hypersensitivity* (see also *type IV hypersensitivity reaction*). The term hypersensitivity implies a heightened reactivity to antigen but it is difficult to define all hypersensitivity reactions, particularly cell-mediated reactions, in such terms.

hypervariable region (HVR; complementarity determining region; CDR) Within the *variable region* of the *heavy chains* and *light chains* of *immunoglobulin* molecules, residues in certain positions show much higher variability from one molecule to another than do residues at other positions (*framework regions*). These hypervariable residues are situated at the bends of loops of the V region (variable region) *domain* which protrude into the *antigen-binding site*, where they are available for binding to the *epitope*. They are, therefore, partly but not wholly responsible for the specificity of the antigen-binding site and also the *idiotypic* variations between immunoglobulins secreted by different clones of cells. There are three hypervariable regions within the variable region of both heavy and light chain.

hypocomplementaemia Any condition in which serum *complement* levels are low. Seen in conditions where *in vivo complement activation* by *immune complexes* is sufficient to depress *serum* levels, e.g. the active phases of proliferative *glomerulonephritis*, *serum sickness*, systemic lupus erythematosus (*SLE*). Levels may also be low in any protein deficiency state.

hypogammaglobulinaemia   Lowered serum *immunoglobulin* (*gamma globulin*) level. May be physiological in neonates or follow increased protein loss or decreased immunoglobulin production. It is also characteristic of *antibody deficiency syndromes*, either familial (e.g. *X-linked agammaglobulinaemia*) or following replacement of *lymphoid tissues* by *lymphoma*, leukaemia, etc.

hyposensitization   (allergen desensitization or Rush desensitization in N. American literature) Administration of a graded series of doses of an *allergen* to subjects suffering from *immediate hypersensitivity* to it, in order to reduce the likelihood of future reactions on casual contact with that allergen. The theory is that the allergen (*antigen*) provokes the production of large amounts of *IgG* (as *blocking antibody*[2]). This IgG either has a direct effect by inhibiting further *IgE* synthesis, or combines with the allergen and prevents the latter from combining with IgE on the surface of *mast cells*. Its practice is restricted, in the UK by the Committee on Safety of Medicines, to use for, mainly, *hay fever* and bee and wasp sting sensitivity; never for asthma. Must be supervised by experts with resuscitation facilities.

I

I-K See *immunoconglutinin*.

I region A region within the *major histocompatibility complex*. The involvement of the products of this region in many aspects of the *immunological response* gave it the general name 'I = immune' region. In the mouse five separate groups of genes are recognized (see *H-2 histocompatibility system*), $A\alpha$, $A\beta$, $E\alpha$, $E\beta$, and $E\beta2$; the equivalents in man (see *HLA histocompatibility system*) are the HLA, DP, DQ and DR regions. See also *H-2I region*.

Ia antigens Also known as *class II MHC antigens*.

iC3b The inactivated form of *C3b*. Often also referred to as C3bi. Although 'inactivated' it binds to *CR3* and *CR4* (though not to *CR1*) and can activate cell function through these receptors. Since it, like C3b, can coat particles, it acts as an *opsonin*. It does not participate in *immune cytolysis* or *alternative pathway* activation.

ICAM-1, -2, -3 (intercellular adhesion molecules) A group of *Type I transmembrane proteins* within the *Ig superfamily*, having a variable number of *constant region*-like domains, and which bind to the β_2 (*leucocyte*) integrins (see *integrin superfamily*). They are important mediators of adhesion of leucocytes to vascular endothelium and to one another, e.g. in clustering of *lymphocytes* round *accessory cells* in induction of an *immune response*. The following molecules have been identified:

(a) **ICAM-1** (CD54) Five Ig domains. The molecule has a wide cellular distribution, is found in low levels on normal vascular endothelium and expression is increased on exposure of the endothelium to activators such as *lipopolysaccharide*, *IL-1* or *TNF-α*. It is found on normal lymphocytes and, again, expression is increased on activation. ICAM-1 binds to the β_2 integrins, *LFA-1* (*CD11a/CD18*) and Mac-1/*CR3* (*CD11b/CD18*). Binding to LFA-1 is an important enhancing step in lymphocyte activation.

(b) **ICAM-2** (CD102) Two Ig domains. Is constitutively expressed on resting vascular endothelium and resting lymphocytes and *monocytes* but not *neutrophil leucocytes*. Its expression is not increased by cell activation. Binds to LFA-1 but not to Mac-1/CR3.

(c) **ICAM-3** (CD50) Five Ig domains. Not expressed on vascular endothelium but highly expressed on resting leucocytes of all types. Binds to LFA-1. See also Table A2.

IDDM See *insulin dependent diabetes mellitus*.

identity, reaction of See *reaction of identity*.

idiopathic thrombocytopenic purpura Human disease characterized by haemorrhagic tendency and purpura (small haemorrhages into the skin) associated with low blood *platelet* count. Associated with the presence of *autoantibodies* against platelets in the *serum*.

idiotope (idiotypic determinant) *Immunoglobulins* are immunogenic, just like any other protein molecule and *antibodies* can be made against any region of the molecule (see also *idiotype*, *allotype*). An idiotope is an *epitope* in the *variable region* of an immunoglobulin that is characteristic of the immunoglobulin molecules produced by a single *B cell* clone, or a small number of clones. It may be present in the *antigen-binding site* or outside it.

idiotype Set of one or more *idiotopes* (q.v.) by which a clone of *immunoglobu-*

lin-forming cells can be distinguished from other clones. Some, known as individual, or private, idiotypes, appear to be unique to individuals. Others, known as inherited, public, or cross reacting idiotypes, are found in many members of the same animal species and even, in some cases, in more than one species.

idiotypic determinant See *idiotope*.

IFN-α, -β (alpha-interferon and beta-interferon; Type I interferons) Two related proteins originally identified as being released by cells in response to viral infection. When the released interferons are bound by other cells replication of the virus within the latter is inhibited. This activity is species-specific, but non-specific in its spectrum of antiviral activity in that virtually all viruses are susceptible to their action. IFN-α was first known as *leucocyte* interferon since it is made by *mononuclear phagocytes*. There are at least 22 protein variants. IFN-β was known as fibroblast interferon. There is only a single form of IFN-β. Both bind to a common *receptor* present on many cells. Both share some sequence homology, but both are unrelated to *IFN-γ* (Type II interferon) and viruses do not induce formation of the latter. The IFN-γ receptor is also different. Note that the protein formerly known as IFN-β$_2$ is now known as *IL-6*.

IFN-γ (gamma-interferon) A *cytokine* produced by activated *T cells* and by *NK cells* which is a major *macrophage* activating factor since it induces *class II MHC antigen* expression and enhances killing of intracellular pathogens by macrophages. It enhances expression of *class I MHC antigen* and class II MHC antigen on many cells, including NK cells and *B cells*, for both of which it is a differentiation factor. IFN-γ release is particularly associated with the T_H1 *cell* subset of *CD4*-positive T cells and drives the *cell-mediated immune* response, but it is also made by *CD8*+ T cells. It binds with high *affinity* to a receptor (CDw119, see Table C1) present on many cells. Binding is species-specific and additional membrane molecules are required for an effective signal to be transduced. IFN-γ has antiviral activity but has little sequence homology with *IFN-α* or *IFN-β* and these latter are more potent antiviral agents than IFN-γ. IFN-γ is cytostatic for many cells; it also activates *neutrophil leucocytes* and causes expression of vascular endothelial adhesion molecules.

Ig Abbreviation for *immunoglobulin*.

Ig-α, Ig-β See *CD79*.

Ig superfamily (immunoglobulin superfamily) A *superfamily* of cell membrane proteins which have in common the presence of extracellular domains (see *immunoglobulin domain*) with an immunoglobulin *constant region* or *variable region*-like structure, though most lack the polymorphism characteristic of *immunoglobulin*. Some proteins carry many such domains, e.g. *CD31* has six; others few, e.g. *Thy-1* has only one. This is by far the largest of the membrane protein superfamilies and numerous examples are cited in this Dictionary, e.g. in the list of CD molecules. The diversity of immunoglobulin-like structures is assumed to result from evolution from a primordial immunoglobulin domain.

IgA The major *immunoglobulin* of the external secretions (intestinal fluids, saliva, bronchial secretions, etc.) in man where it is found as a dimer linked to a *secretory piece* (transport piece) q.v. Also present in *serum* (concentration 1.5–4.0 mg/ml) as a monomer and in polymeric forms (dimer, trimer, tetramer). MW of monomer 170 kD, dimer in secretions MW 400 kD. Does not cross human placenta. Present in human *colostrum* and milk, but is not major colostral immunoglobulin of sow, cow or ewe. Does not activate *complement* except in presence of *lysozyme* or, in polymerized form, via the *alternative pathway*. Synthesis primarily in *lymphoid tissues* of gut, respiratory tract and Harderian gland (tear gland) of the bird. Secretory form probably not derived from serum but synthesized locally. Two subclasses in man (see *immunoglobulin subclass*). Forms major specific humoral defence mechanism on mucosal surfaces. See Figure I1.

IgA deficiency A common selective *immunodeficiency* (1:700 of UK or USA populations) characterized by low *serum* levels of *IgA* and normal levels of other *immunoglobulins*. In many cases, there is no clinical abnormality. However IgA deficient persons may make anti-IgA *antibodies* if they receive blood transfusions. Some patients have recurrent infections and there is an increased incidence of *autoimmune diseases* such as *SLE* or *rheumatoid arthritis*.

IgA Fc receptor See *Fcα receptor*.

IgD *Immunoglobulin* present in low concentration in human *serum* (0.03–0.4 mg/ml). MW 184 kD. Confined to intravascular space. Low concentration partly attributable to rapid catabolism, i.e. short half-life. Present in large quantities as *membrane immunoglobulin* on the surface of *B lymphocytes* where it acts, with membrane *IgM* (see *membrane immunoglobulin*), as a *receptor* for *antigen*.

IgE The main *immunoglobulin* associated with *immediate hypersensitivity* (*type I hypersensitivity reaction*). Present in *serum* in very low concentration (20–500 ng/ml) but elevated in *atopic* individuals who suffer from *asthma* or *hay fever*, and also in persons infected with intestinal helminths. High *affinity* for FcεRI (see *Fcε receptors*) on the surface of *mast cells*. MW 188 kD. High carbohydrate content (11%). Present in external secretions. Major sites of synthesis are *lymphoid tissues* of the gut and respiratory tract.

IgE Fc receptor See *Fcε receptors*.

IgG The major *immunoglobulin* in the *serum* of man. Homologous immunoglobulins are found in most species from amphibians upwards, but are not present in fish. Molecular weight of human IgG 150 kD. There are four subclasses in man *IgG1, IgG2, IgG3* and *IgG4* but the number varies in other species (see *immunoglobulin subclass*). Normal serum concentration in man 8–16 mg/ml. IgG1, 2 and 3 fix *complement* by the *classical complement pathway* with different efficiencies, but not IgG4. All four subclasses are able to cross the human placenta. See Figure I2.

IgG Fc receptor See *Fcγ receptors*.

IgG subclass deficiencies A variable group of *immunoglobulin* deficiency states often associated with recurrent

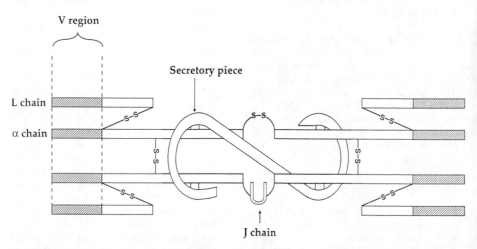

Figure I1. IgA. A schematic diagram of human IgA1. In human IgA2m(1) and mouse IgA, the L chains are not linked to the α chains by disulphide bridges, as shown here, but to each other as an L₂ dimer. The precise arrangement of the disulphide bridges linking J chain and secretory piece to the α chains is not certain.

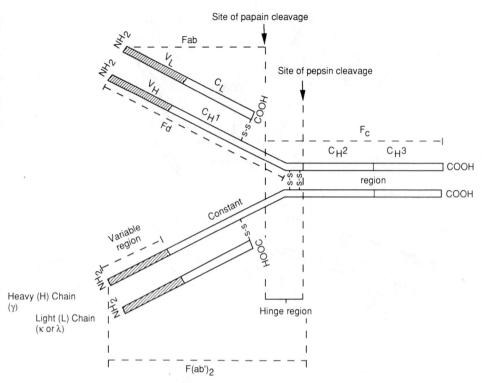

Figure I2. IgG. A schematic diagram of human IgG1 showing the sites of cleavage by proteolytic enzymes and the resulting fragments.

infections. *IgG2* (see *IgG*) deficiency predisposes to severe infections by bacteria with carbohydrate capsules such as *Streptococcus pneumoniae* or *Haemophilus influenzae*. It is sometimes found together with deficiency of *IgA* and *IgG4*.

IgG1, IgG2, IgG3, IgG4 The *immunoglobulin subclasses* of human *IgG* (q.v. for details of differences). A similar nomenclature is used for IgG subclasses in other species, e.g. in the mouse IgG1, IgG2a, IgG2b and IgG3.

Ig_κ locus The region of the genome containing all the *exons* (L_p, V, J, $C_κ$) coding for κ *light chains*.

Ig_λ locus The region of the genome containing all the *exons* (L_p, V, J, $C_λ$) coding for λ *light chains*.

IgM High molecular weight (970 kD) *immunoglobulin*. Phylogenetically the

most primitive immunoglobulin, present in all vertebrates from lamprey upwards. In mammals it is mainly in the form of a cyclic pentamer of five basic four chain units of two *heavy chains* and two *light chains* linked by disulphide bonds. A monomeric form is found on the surface of *B lymphocytes* (Figure C3). In other species the predominant form may be a monomer (e.g. dogfish) tetramer (e.g. carp) or hexamer (*Xenopus*). Heavy (μ) chain larger than that of other immunoglobulins (MW 70 kD). High carbohydrate content. Activates *complement*. Does not cross placenta in man but may in certain other species (e.g. rabbit). Antibody activity usually destroyed by reduction of intersubunit disulphide bonds. Normal *serum* concentration in man is 0.5–2.0 mg/ml. See Figure I3.

Ii See *invariant chain*.

IL Abbreviation for *interleukin*.

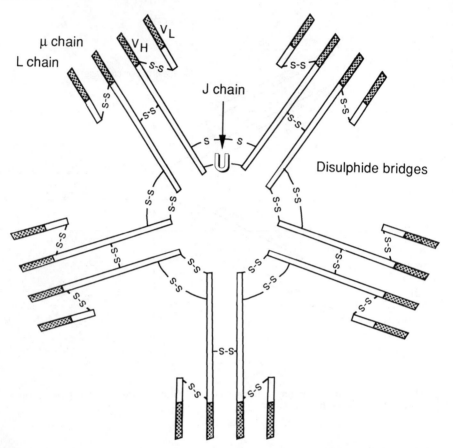

Figure I3. IgM. A schematic diagram of human IgM. The outer inter-subunit disulphide bridges are absent in mouse IgM.

IL-1 The designation, IL-1, includes two related proteins, IL-1α and IL-1β, produced by separate genes in the same cluster. Both are 17 kD proteins and both are capable of binding to the same cell surface *receptors*. IL-1α and β share many functions. IL-1 is made by many cell types, but particularly by *mononuclear phagocytes* after activation with microbial products such as *lipopolysaccharide*. It is not produced by unactivated cells. It is an inflammatory *cytokine* which induces fever (i.e. is an endogenous pyrogen), increases adhesion molecule expression by vascular endothelium, and causes neutrophilia (see *neutrophil leucocyte*), hypotension and synthesis of *acute phase reactants*. It was originally described as a *T lymphocyte* activating factor and it co-stimulates activation of some *CD4+* T cells. In *primary immune responses* it may activate T cells by enhancing the *accessory cell* function of *dendritic cells*. It activates *macrophages* to produce more IL-1 as well as to produce *TNF-α* and *IL-6*. It induces collagenase release implicated in cartilage destruction. Many of its effects are related to its ability to cause *prostaglandin* release (also *PAF* and *nitric oxide*) in cells to which it binds. Functions are similar to those of *TNF-α* and it is produced in response to similar stimuli.

IL-1R (IL-1 receptor; CDw121) There are two forms of IL-1R, type I (CDw121a, see Table C1) found on *T* cells, *mononuclear phagocytes*, endothelial cells and many other cell types, and type II (CDw121b, see Table C1) found on *B cells* and mononuclear phagocytes. They are both *Type I transmembrane proteins* of the *Ig superfamily* and both bind IL-1α and IL-1β (see *IL-1*) with high *affinity*, but only type I IL-1R transduces a signal.

IL-1R antagonist (IL-1 receptor antagonist) A protein closely related to *IL-1* and derived from the same gene cluster, which competes with IL-1 for both forms of *IL-1R* (IL-1 receptors) and, since it does not activate the cells it binds to, blocks the functions of IL-1. It is thus an important inflammatory regulator. It is made by *macrophages*, *neutrophil leucocytes* and vascular endothelial cells. *IL-4* and *IL-10* induce synthesis of IL-1R antagonist by macrophages and inhibit synthesis of IL-1.

IL-2 A *cytokine* whose major function is in regulation of the *immune response*. It is synthesized primarily by *helper T lymphocytes* following *T cell* recognition of *class II MHC* (associated) *antigen* and by agents such as *mitogens* that mimic that recognition. IL-2 activates growth and proliferation of T lymphocytes and is required for them to pass from the G1 to the S phase of the cell cycle. IL-2 synthesis and release is a characteristic of the T_H1 *cell* subset, and drives the immune response towards CMI (*cell-mediated immunity*) responses such as *delayed-type hypersensitivity*. It is required to initiate all T cell responses and is essential for the growth of *CD8+* cells. It also enhances *NK cell* function and is a growth factor for *germinal centre* B cells but not for nongerminal centre *B cells*.

IL-2R (IL-2 receptor) A receptor for *IL-2* found on *T cells, B cells, NK cells* and *monocytes*. Consists of at least three subunits, α, β and γ. All three are *Type I transmembrane proteins*, the α subunit belongs to the *SCR superfamily*, and the β and γ subunits have *cytokine receptor superfamily* domains. IL-2Rα (*CD25*) is lacking on resting T cells and NK cells but is expressed following activation. IL-2 binds with low *affinity* to the isolated

α subunit. IL-2Rβ (*CD122*) is present on both resting and activated *lymphocytes* and associates closely with IL-2Rγ. IL-2Rγ is also found on *IL-4R* and IL-7R and γ-chain gene mutations are found in some cases of X-linked *SCID*. IL-2 binds with intermediate affinity to cells bearing β and γ, and with high affinity to cells bearing α, β and γ. On binding of IL-2 the cytoplasmic regions of β and γ dimerize and this is essential for transmission of a signal. Binding of IL-2 to IL-2R stimulates growth and proliferation of T cells, NK cells, and B cells *inter alia*.

IL-3 A *haemopoietic growth factor*, derived chiefly from *T cells*, that stimulates proliferation and differentiation of *bone marrow* pluripotential *stem cells* and lineage-committed precursors. Lineage-restricted factors such as *GM-CSF*, *M-CSF*, etc. are required for the full differentiation of the latter. Also activates *mucosal mast cells* and *pre-B lymphocytes*.

IL-3R A heterodimeric *Type I transmembrane protein* of the *cytokine receptor (haemopoietic growth factor) superfamily*. Found on *bone marrow* pluripotential *stem cells* and on committed stem cells of the *myeloid cell series* lineage, *eosinophil leucocyte* and *basophil leucocyte* precursors, *mast cell* precursors and precursors of cells other than those of the immune system. Has an α chain unique to IL-3R and a β chain common to IL-3R, *IL-5R* and *GM-CSFR*. *IL-3* binds to the isolated α chain with low *affinity* and to the α,β dimer with high affinity.

IL-4 A *cytokine* derived from activated *T lymphocytes* (see *activated lymphocyte*); previously known as B cell growth factor I. It activates *B cells* very early in growth and allows B cells activated by *antigen*, anti *IgM* or *lipopolysaccharide* to move into the G1 phase of the cell cycle. It enhances *class II MHC antigen* expression and expression of *CD23* (FcεRII) in B cells and induces *isotype switching* to IgG1 (mouse) and *IgE*. It also enhances class II MHC antigen expression in *mononuclear phagocytes*, but has an inhibitory effect on inflammatory cytokine release (i.e. *IL-1, TNF, IL-8*) and on the microbicidal activity of these cells. It also activates *cytotoxic T lymphocytes*. IL-4 is regarded as the typical cytokine made by T_H2 *cells*, being essential for the development of these cells and driving the *immune response* towards *humoral immunity* and *antibody* production.

IL-4R (CDw124) A *Type I transmembrane protein* of the *cytokine receptor superfamily*, found on many cell types including *pre-B lymphocytes*, mature *B cells, T cells, macrophages* and others. While *IL-4* binding to the membrane receptor activates the functions listed for IL-4, there is a soluble form of IL-4R which inhibits IL-4 mediated functions.

IL-5 A T_H2 *cell*-derived *cytokine* that induces activation and differentiation of *eosinophil leucocytes* and differentiation of activated mouse *B cells* to become *antibody*-secreting cells (IL-5 acting later than *IL-4* induces *isotype switching* to *IgA*). IL-5 production is increased in helminthic diseases characterized by *eosinophilia* and eosinophil activation. IL-5 is also an activator of *basophil leucocytes*.

IL-5R A heterodimeric *Type I transmembrane protein* with a unique α chain associated with a β chain which is common to the *IL-5, IL-3* and *GM-CSF* receptors. Both chains contain *cytokine receptor superfamily* domains and fibronectin-like domains. Found on *eosinophil leucocytes, basophil leucocytes* and murine *B cells*.

IL-6 (previously called interferon-β_2) A *cytokine* of particular importance in inflammatory reactions. It is produced by many cell types including *mononuclear phagocytes, T* and *B lymphocytes*, vascular endothelium and numerous cells outside the immune system. IL-6 production is enhanced by inflammatory signals, e.g. *lipopolysaccharide, IL-1* and *TNF*. Activities include B cell differentiation to *antibody* secreting cells (acting later than *IL-4*); growth of and IL-2 production by T cells; effects on growth of *bone marrow* stem cells;

stimulation of *acute phase reactant* release, and many others.

IL-6R A heterodimeric *Type I transmembrane protein* with an α chain (CD126, see Table C1) and a β chain (CDw130, see Table C1), both of which contain *immunoglobulin*-like domains, *cytokine receptor superfamily* domains and fibronectin-like domains. Both chains are required to bind *IL-6* strongly as the isolated α chain binds weakly and the β chain not at all. Found on activated *B cells* and many other cell types. A soluble form exists as a result of proteolytic cleavage of membrane IL-6R.

IL-7 A *cytokine* originally derived from *bone marrow* stromal cells and identified as a proliferation factor for *pre-B lymphocytes*. It also has effects on growth and proliferation of *thymocytes* and *T cells* including *cytotoxic T lymphocytes*. Its receptor is a *Type I transmembrane protein* not related to the major superfamilies and found on the various lymphocytes mentioned above.

IL-8 (NAP-1) An α-*chemokine* and the first member of the chemokine family to be described. IL-8 is a *neutrophil leucocyte* chemotactic factor (see *chemotaxis*) and activates other neutrophil functions including adhesion and microbicidal activity. Also has chemotactic activity for activated *T lymphocytes* (see *activated lymphocyte*); activity for *basophil leucocytes* has been reported. Normally found as a 14 kD homodimer. Made in large amounts by *macrophages*, endothelial cells and other cells following inflammatory stimulation.

IL-8R (CDw128) See *chemokine receptors*.

IL-9 A *cytokine* derived from activated *T cells* (see *activated lymphocyte*) that supports growth and proliferation of T cells and, with other cytokines, enhances growth of *bone marrow*-derived *mast cells*.

IL-10 A *cytokine* produced by *T lymphocytes*, especially T_H2 *cells*, as well as by *mononuclear phagocytes*, activated *B cells* (see *activated lymphocytes*) and others. It suppresses cytokine release and *class II MHC antigen* expression by mononuclear phagocytes, and inhibits *antigen presentation* to T_H1 *cells*, and thus probably diminishes *delayed-type hypersensitivity* responses. Conversely it enhances class II MHC antigen expression on B cells and their proliferation and differentiation, as well as the proliferation of *thymocytes* and *mast cells*.

IL-11 A *haemopoietic growth factor* with growth and proliferative effects on *stem cells* of various lineages in the *bone marrow* as well as on non-bone marrow derived cells. Made chiefly by fibroblasts and fibroblast-like cells. Functionally similar to *IL-6*.

IL-12 A heterodimeric *cytokine* (formerly known as *NK cell* stimulating factor) which activates NK cells and *T cells*. One of its chains has homology with *IL-6*, the other with the IL-6 receptor (*IL-6R*). IL-12 is made chiefly by *macrophages* and other *accessory cells*. It causes proliferation and enhances the cytotoxicity of both NK cells and *CD8+ cytotoxic T lymphocytes*. It polarizes the *immune response* towards T_H1 *cells*, by enhancing **IFN-γ** production and inducing macrophage activation. It is thus a protective cytokine in infections by intracellular pathogens.

IL-13 An *IL-4*-like *cytokine* secreted by activated T cells (see *activated lymphocytes*). The IL-13 gene is close to the gene for IL-4 and there is sequence homology between the two proteins. IL-13, like IL-4, is an activator of *B cell* growth early in the cell cycle. Like IL-4, it is both an inhibitor of microbicidal activity and cytokine release by *mononuclear phagocytes* and an enhancer of *antigen presentation* by these cells.

IL-14 A *B cell* growth factor, derived from *T lymphocytes* or B cell lines, that induces proliferation of activated, but not resting, B cells.

IL-15 A *cytokine* produced by many cell types with similar effects to *IL-2* as an activator of *T cell* proliferation and effector function. *Chemoattractant* for T lymphocytes. It does not share sequence homology with IL-2 but has a similar predicted three-dimensional structure and binds to *IL-2R*.

immediate hypersensitivity *IgE* antibody-mediated *hypersensitivity* characterized by lesions resulting from release of *histamine* and other vasoactive substances (synonym *type 1 hypersensitivity reaction*). IgE *antibody* fixes to *basophil leucocytes* and, especially, to *mast cells* in the tissues. On combination of this antibody with *antigen* the cells rapidly release their vasoactive substances. Symptoms or lesions appear from a few seconds to 30 minutes after contact with the antigen, hence name. IgE is detected by *skin tests* and the *radioallergosorbent test* (RAST) in man and *passive cutaneous anaphylaxis* in animals. For examples see *anaphylaxis, hay fever, asthma* and *urticaria*.

immobilization test Technique for the detection and/or titration of *antibody* against a motile bacterium or protozoon, etc. by observing the effect of antibody in inhibiting movement. This inhibition may be caused by: (a) adhesion together (in effect *agglutination*) of the cilia or flagella of organisms, e.g. *Trichomonas fetus, Paramoecium* spp., or motile bacteria; or (b) damage to the cell wall in the presence of *complement* as in *Treponema pallidum* immobilization test (the causative organism of syphilis).

immune (1) Protected against disease either by (a) specific or (b) non-specific mechanism; e.g. in (a) those who have been *vaccinated* against or have recovered from poliomyelitis are immune to it, and in (b) all humans are immune to canine distemper. (2) A state in which, following contact with *antigen* the tissues show a specific alteration in their reactivity to subsequent doses of that antigen, inasmuch as they now exhibit a response of *humoral immunity*, or *cell-mediated immunity* against it.

immune adherence Adherence of *immune complexes* or *antibody* coated bacteria, etc. to primate erythrocytes, rabbit *platelets, macrophages* and *polymorphonuclear leucocytes* (polymorphs). In the case of macrophages and polymorphs immune adherence stimulates *phagocytosis*. The phenomenon is *complement*-dependent and occurs when *C3* is bound and is a property of *C3b* and C4b (see *C4*). May be used as sensitive detector system for *complement fixing antibody*.

immune clearance See *immune elimination*.

immune complex A macromolecular complex of *antigen* and *antibody* molecules bound specifically together. May be present in soluble form especially in *antigen excess* or as a precipitate especially at *optimal proportions*. *Complement* components may be bound by immune complexes. Important in pathogenesis of certain *hypersensitivity* reactions, see *Arthus reaction* (*type III hypersensitivity reaction*). See also *immune complex disease, serum sickness, glomerulonephritis*.

immune complex disease Tissue damage mediated by *immune complexes*, especially seen in human and experimental *glomerulonephritis*. Essentially *hypersensitivity* of *Arthus reaction* type (*type III hypersensitivity reaction*) q.v. See also *serum sickness, Masugi nephritis and Goodpasture's syndrome*.

immune cytolysis (1) Lysis of cells by *antibody* in the presence of *complement*. Term usually used of cells other than erythrocytes, cf. *immune haemolysis*. (2) Lysis of target cells by *cytotoxic T lymphocytes* or other cytotoxic cells, e.g. *NK cells*.

immune elimination (1) Exponential elimination of *antigen* from the body as a result of removal and destruction by *antibodies* and/or *effector cells*. This commences a few days after the first administration of the antigen and radiolabelled antigens can be shown to be eliminated from the circulation much more rapidly in *immune²* than in *non-immune animals*. (2) Technique used to measure the antibody response by following the rate of removal of a labelled antigen from the circulation of an *immunized²* animal.

immune exclusion Process by which entry of *antigen* into the body is prevented by a specific *immune response* directed at the antigen. The term is most frequently applied to the regulation of antigen absorption by mucosal surfaces. It is also used to describe a mechanism by which helminth larvae are prevented from becoming established in the gut.

immune haemolysis *Complement*-dependent mechanism by which fresh *serum* (i.e. containing complement) lyses erythrocytes coated with anti erythrocyte *antibody*, i.e. a *haemolytic system*.

immune response The specific response to *antigen*. Thus includes the responses of *cell-mediated immunity, humoral immunity* and, in its widest sense *immunological tolerance* though, strictly speaking, the latter is a state of specific *immunological unresponsiveness*.

immune serum *Antiserum* especially in context of *protective immunity*.

immune state (1) The state of responsiveness of a host to any antigen, e.g. tolerant (see *immunological tolerance*), non-immune (see *non-immune animal*), *immune¹,²*, etc. (2) Used in a more restricted sense in prophylactic *immunization²* to describe the degree of *protective immunity* which an individual possesses against a pathogenic organism, e.g. solid immunity, partial immunity, etc.

immune tolerance See *immunological tolerance*.

immunity (1) Synonyms: *protective immunity* and functional immunity. Non-susceptibility to the invasive or pathogenic effects of foreign organisms or to the toxic effects of antigenic substances (see *antigen*). See also *active immunity, passive immunity* and *non-specific immunity*. (2) State of heightened responsiveness to antigen, such that antigen is bound or eliminated more rapidly than in the non-immune state (see *non-immune animal*); thus inclusive of all types of *humoral immun-*

ity and *cell-mediated immunity* but not of *immunological tolerance.*

immunity deficiency syndrome See *immunodeficiency.*

immunization (1) Administration of *antigen* in order to produce an *immune response* to that antigen. (2) In clinical contexts the term is used more specifically to mean administration either of antigen to produce *active immunity* or, of *antibody* to produce *passive immunity,* in order to confer protection against harmful effects of antigenic substances or organisms.

immunize See *immunization.*

immunoblotting (western blotting) A technique for the analysis and identification of protein *antigens.* The proteins are separated by *polyacrylamide gel electrophoresis* and then transferred electrophoretically to a membrane of nitrocellulose or other material to which the proteins bind in a pattern identical to that originally in the gel (the 'blot'). Bands of antigen bound to the nitrocellulose are detected by overlaying with *antibody* followed by anti *immunoglobulin* or *protein A* labelled with a radioisotope, fluorescent dye or enzyme (e.g. horseradish peroxidase or alkaline phosphatase). The advantages of this technique are that the antigens are exposed on the surface of the membrane and are immobilized, whereas direct overlay of the gel with antibody results in lower sensitivity, due to the slow penetration of the gel by antibody, and loss of resolution due to diffusion of the antigen. Many variations exist including the use of other gel electrophoresis systems, non-electrophoretic transfer methods and antibody-coated membrane to bind selectively the antigen of interest. See also *reverse immunoblotting.*

immunoconglutinin *Autoantibody* against fixed *complement* components, especially *C3,* also *C4,* i.e. *C3b* and C4b (see C4). Serum immunoconglutinin levels reflect extent of *complement fixation* by *in vivo immunological reactions* and are raised in many bacterial, viral and parasitic infections and *autoimmune*

diseases. Not to be confused with *conglutinin* q.v.

immunodeficiency Any condition in which a deficiency of *humoral immunity* or *cell-mediated immunity* exists. Examples are: *severe combined immunodeficiency syndrome, cell-mediated immunity deficiency syndromes, X-linked agammaglobulinaemia, antibody deficiency syndrome, inter alia.*

immunodiffusion See *gel diffusion test.*

immunodominance An immunodominant portion of an *epitope* is a part that contributes a disproportionately large portion of the binding energy. Many *haptens* are immunodominant.

immunoelectrophoresis Technique in which proteins are first separated by electrophoresis and then allowed to react with an *antiserum* so that a pattern of *precipitation* arcs is developed. Proteins are thus characterized by (a) electrophoretic mobility; and (b) *antigenic* character. Used for the analysis of complex mixtures such as *serum.*

immunoferritin technique The electron microscopic visualization of *epitopes* using ferritin-labelled *antibody* applied directly to the specimen, or a ferritin-labelled antiglobulin (see *antiglobulin test*) may be used for indirect techniques analogous to those used in *indirect immunofluorescence.*

immunofluorescence Technique in which *antigen* or *antibody* is conjugated to a *fluorochrome* and then allowed to react with its corresponding antibody or antigen in a tissue section or cell suspension. The location of tissue antibodies or antigens is then determined by microscopic observation, or the proportion of fluorescent cells in a cell population measured using a *fluorescence activated cell sorter.* For the principal ways in which the technique is applied see *direct immunofluorescence, indirect immunofluorescence, sandwich immunofluorescence* and *double layer immunofluorescence.*

immunogen A substance that when introduced into the body stimulates *humoral immunity* or *cell-mediated immunity* as opposed to *immunological tolerance*.

immunogenic Capable of inducing *humoral immunity* or *cell-mediated immunity* but not *immunological tolerance*. Cf. *tolerogenic*.

immunogenicity The potential of an *antigen* (or *immunogen*) to stimulate an *immune response*.

immunoglobulin Member of a family of proteins each made up of *light chains* and *heavy chains* linked together by disulphide bonds. The members are divided into *immunoglobulin classes* and *immunoglobulin subclasses* (q.v.) determined by the amino acid sequence of their heavy chains. Most mammals have five immunoglobulin classes (*IgM*, *IgG*, *IgA*, *IgD*, *IgE*), although lower organisms have fewer, e.g. the cartilaginous fishes have only one immunoglobulin closely related to IgM. All *antibodies* are immunoglobulins; however, it is not certain that all immunoglobulin molecules function as antibodies. Present in *serum* and other body fluids. On electrophoresis show γ or β mobility relative to other serum proteins. See Table I1 and Figures I1, I2 and I3.

immunoglobulin A See *IgA*.

immunoglobulin class The group into which an *immunoglobulin* is placed by virtue of the amino acid sequence of the *constant region* of its *heavy chain* which distinguishes it from the other classes; the chains being named with the Greek letter equivalent for each class. The γ chain of *IgG* for instance, differs in the amino acid sequence of its constant region from that of the heavy chains of the other immunoglobulin classes. *IgA*, *IgD*, *IgE*, IgG and *IgM* are immunoglobulin classes distinguishable respectively by their possession of α, δ, ε, γ and μ chains. It is the heavy chain constant region that determines the overall structure and properties of the immunoglobulin molecule, viz. number of *domains*, monomeric/polymeric structure, *complement* activation, etc. See Table I1.

immunoglobulin D See *IgD*.

immunoglobulin domain The three-dimensional structure formed by a single *homology region* of the *heavy chain* or *light chain* of an *immunoglobulin*, i.e. V_L region, C_L, V_H region, C_H1–C_H4. Each homology region is folded into a similar three-dimensional shape which is believed to be shared by homology regions present in other members of the *Ig superfamily*. All members of the Ig superfamily are characterized by the presence of *domains* resembling the variable or constant domains of immunoglobulin.

immunoglobulin E See *IgE*.

immunoglobulin G See *IgG*.

immunoglobulin gene See Figures I4 and I5.

immunoglobulin M See *IgM*.

immunoglobulin subclass Subdivision within each *immunoglobulin class*, based on structural and antigenic differences in their *heavy chains*. Thus human *IgG* has four subclasses: *IgG1*, *IgG2*, *IgG3* and *IgG4*. The γ chains (γ1, γ2, γ3 and γ4) of the subclasses show closer sequence homology to each other than to the heavy chains of the other immunoglobulin classes. The subclasses differ structurally from one another, e.g. IgG1 and IgG4 have two inter-heavy chain disulphide bonds in the *hinge region*, IgG2 has four and IgG3 has 11. They also differ functionally, e.g. IgG1, 2 and 3 activate *complement* whereas IgG4 does not. Human *IgA* has two subclasses, IgA1 and IgA2. Immunoglobulins of other species also show subclass differences, e.g. mouse IgG1, IgG2a, IgG2b and IgG3.

immunoglobulin superfamily See *Ig superfamily*.

immunogold labelling A technique in which *antibody* is tagged with spheres of colloidal gold. Since gold is electron-

Table I1. Characteristics of the human immunoglobulins

Character	IgG	IgA	IgM	IgD	IgE
Electrophoretic mobility	γ_2-γ_1	γ_1 to β	γ_1	γ_1	γ_1
Molecular weight (kD)	150	170 in serum (forms polymers) Dimer in secretions 398	970	184	188
Sedimentation coefficient (approx.)	7S	7S (monomer) 11S (dimer)	19S	7S	8S
Concentration in human serum (mg/ml)	8–16	1.5–4.0	0.5–2.0	0.03–0.4	20–500 ng/ml
Per cent of total Ig in plasma pool	78–85	7–15	5–10	0–0.1	0.002–0.003
Catabolic rate as per cent of intravascular pool per day	4–7	14–34	14–25	18–60	
Valency	2	2 (monomer) 4 (dimer)	5–10	2	2
Heavy chain type	γ	α	μ	δ	ε
Light chain type	κ and λ	κ and λ	κ and λ	κ and λ	κ and λ
Where found	Plasma, tissue fluids	External secretions (e.g. saliva, milk) Plasma	Plasma	Plasma	Plasma, Secretions
Complement activation (classical pathway)	Yes, sub-classes IgG1, -2 and -3	No (in absence of lysozyme)	Yes	No	No
Placental transfer	Yes	No	No	No	No

dense, the antibody can be precisely located in or on cells by electron microscopy. The technique is specially useful for locating *antigens*. It can also be used in light microscopy. Spheres of different sizes can be tagged to different antibodies allowing visualization of more than one antigen in the same preparation (*double labelling*).

immunological Referring to *specific immunity*, e.g. as in *immunological tolerance*, or to the study of immunology, e.g. immunological journals.

immunological barrier Anatomical barrier that prevents or attenuates an

immune response against an *antigen*. Examples are: the placenta (prevents *immunological rejection* of mammalian fetus) and the aqueous humour of the eye (allows *alloantigenic* grafts to be made to the anterior chamber).

immunological competence Capacity to produce an *immune response*; used of cells, tissues, etc.

immunological deficiency state Preferred term is *immunodeficiency*.

immunological enhancement An increased rate of tumour growth in animals immunized (see *immunization*)

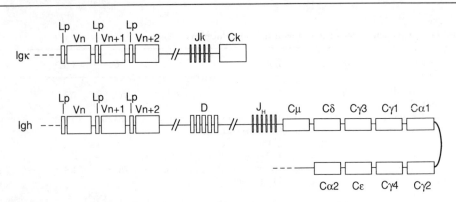

Figure I4. Immunoglobulin gene. Human germline Igκ and Igh loci. Exons are denoted by □ and non-coding regions (introns) by —. The figures are not to scale. The heavy chain constant region genes (Cμ, Cδ, etc.) are divided into separate exons coding for each domain, the hinge region and the membrane tail sequence. A single box is shown for each constant region for simplicity.

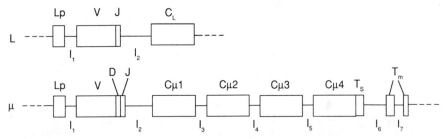

Figure I5. Immunoglobulin gene. The structure of light and heavy chain genes from an IgM-produc-ing cell. L, light chain gene; μ, μ chain gene; Lp, leader peptide exon; V, variable region exon; D, D exon (heavy chain only); J, J exon; C_L, light chain constant region exon; Cμ1–4, μ constant region exons; T_S, tail sequence; T_m, exons coding for the membrane and cytoplasmic tail sequence of the membrane-bound form of μ chain. All coding regions (exons) are shown as blocks. Introns I_1, I_2, etc. are shown as straight lines.

with the *antigens* of the tumour. Seen especially in experimental tumours transplanted to animals which have *antibody* to the tumour. Attributed to the coating of tumour antigens with antibody which prevents access of *cytotoxic T lymphocytes* (agents of *cell-mediated immunity*) to the tumour cells.

immunological inertia A specific depression of *immunity*, other than *immunological tolerance*, towards the *histocompatibility antigens* of a partner in viviparity, i.e. of mother or of fetus.

immunological memory Concept for-mulated to explain the capacity of the immunological system to respond much faster and more powerfully to sub-sequent exposures to an *antigen* than it did at the first exposure.

immunological reaction (1) *In vivo.* Any reaction or response stemming from the contact of *primed* or *unprimed lymphocytes* with, or the combination of *antibody* with, an *antigen*, e.g. cell division, *lymphocyte activation*, anti-body production, induction of *immuno-logical tolerance*, *graft rejection*, *hyper-sensitivity*, etc. (2) *In vitro.* Any measurable change resulting from the combination of antibody with, or response of *primed lymphocytes* to, an antigen, e.g. *precipitation*, virus neu-tralization, etc.

immunological rejection Destruction of foreign cells or tissues inoculated or grafted into a recipient due to a reaction of *specific immunity* against them.

immunological surveillance Postulated continuous monitoring of the cells of the body by its immunological system so that aberrant cells arising by somatic mutation and containing new *antigens* are rapidly destroyed. Suggested by Burnet as control mechanism in prevention of neoplasia.

immunological tolerance The induction of specific non-reactivity of the *lymphoid tissues* to an *antigen* capable in other circumstances of inducing active *cell-mediated* or *humoral immunity*. May follow contact with antigen in fetal or early post-natal life or, in adults, after administration of very high or very low doses of certain antigens. *Immunological reactions[1]* to unrelated antigens are not affected by the induction of tolerance to any given antigen. Tolerance may be due to *anergy, clonal deletion* or active suppression of antigen-specific clones of *T* or *B lymphocytes*.

immunological unresponsiveness Failure to respond to contact with *antigen*. May be specific for a given antigen, as in *immunological tolerance* and *Ir gene* (q.v.) defects, or generalized inasmuch as there is non-specific unresponsiveness to many antigens as, for example in *immunodeficiency* states or following therapy with an *immunosuppressive* agent.

immunophilins Collective name for *cyclophilins* and *FKBPs* q.v.

immunopotentiation Term used for artificial augmentation of the *immune response* in a very general sense. Is thus the opposite of *immunosuppression*. Produced by a wide variety of agents, e.g. *adjuvants*.

immunoprophylaxis The prevention of disease by the use of *vaccines* or *antisera*.

immunosuppression The artificial suppression of *immune responses*. Used to enhance survival of *allografts*. See *cyclosporin A* and *FK506®*.

immunotherapy Treatment of disease by *active immunization* or *passive immunization* or by the use of agents designed to potentiate or suppress the actions of *lymphocytes*.

immunotoxin A toxin conjugated to an *antibody* or antibody fragment. Toxins conjugated to antibodies against specific cell-surface *antigens*, e.g. on tumour cells, can thus be targeted to those cells, e.g. ricin has been conjugated to anti tumour antibodies in an attempt to destroy tumour cells *in vivo*.

in situ **hybridization** Technique for localizing expression of specific genes in tissues. A labelled DNA or RNA probe is added to a tissue section and binds specifically to complementary mRNA. The pattern of labelling then identifies which cells in the tissue express the gene in question.

inactivated vaccine A vaccine containing pathogenic viruses, bacteria or other organisms that are incapable of replication. Viruses are usually inactivated by, e.g. formaldehyde, phenol or β-propiolactone; bacteria by formaldehyde, phenol, acetone or heat. The object is to cause as little damage as possible to the *protective antigens* of the organism. Cf. *attenuated vaccine*.

inactivation (1) Any procedure used to destroy any biological activity. (2) Destruction of *complement* activity in *serum*, e.g. by heating at 56°C for 20 minutes or by treatment with hydrazine, etc. See *heat inactivation*. (3) The use of heat, formaldehyde, phenol, or β-propiolactone to kill a pathogenic virus, bacterium or other organism before preparing an *inactivated vaccine* from it.

inbred strain Experimental animals produced by sequential brother–sister matings. In immunology, the term usually refers to animals in the 20th and subsequent generations of such matings. Such animals are so homogeneous at *histocompatibility loci* that grafts can be freely exchanged between them without provoking *graft rejection*. Note that, due to mutations and evolutionary pressure, sublines of inbred strains kept in different laboratories, may gradually lose syngeneity. Many inbred strains and substrains carry mutations that may be of value in immunological experimentation, see *B/B rat, beige mice, C3H mice, CBA mice, non-obese diabetic mice, NZB mice, NZW mice, MRL-lpr/lpr mice*.

incompatibility Antigenic non-identity between donor and recipient, e.g. in blood transfusion or tissue transplantation, such that harmful reactions may occur when donor material is introduced into the recipient. Examples of such reactions are *transfusion reactions* and *immunological rejection*.

incomplete Freund's adjuvant A *water-in-oil emulsion adjuvant*. Cf. *complete Freund's adjuvant* and note that the incomplete form does not contain mycobacteria.

indirect complement fixation test Test used to detect *antibodies* that do not fix guinea pig *complement*, e.g. avian antibodies. Dilutions of avian *serum* are allowed to react with the antigen. Complement and rabbit antibody to the *antigen* are then added to each dilution. Antigen which has not combined with the avian antibody (in the tube where the latter has been diluted out), is available to combine with the rabbit antibody and in so doing fixes the complement. The extent of fixation is detected by adding a *haemolytic system*. Lysis of the cells indicates that avian antibody was initially present in those tubes.

indirect immunofluorescence A technique for detecting *antibody* or *antigen* in which two or more layers of reagent are used (cf. *direct immunofluorescence*). The first layer is a reagent that will specifically combine with the molecule to be detected. The second layer, conjugated with a *fluorochrome*, is specific for that first layer. Advantages over direct immunofluorescence are that the indirect technique gives a multiplication effect (and hence greater sensitivity) as

more sites for combination are available, also the labelled second reagent can be employed in several systems. Examples are *sandwich immunofluorescence* and *double layer immunofluorescence*. See Figure I6.

inductive phase Period of time that elapses between the administration of an *antigen* and the appearance of a *detectable immune response*. The true inductive phase will be much shorter than this.

infantile sex-linked hypogamma-globulinaemia See *X-linked agamma-globulinaemia*.

infectious mononucleosis (glandular fever) Infectious disease caused by Epstein–Barr virus (EBV) which infects *B lymphocytes*. Characterized by fever, sore throat, and *lymph node* enlargement. Typically there are many large, activated *T lymphocytes* (see *activated lymphocyte*) in the blood, reactive against the EBV-infected B cells. *Antibodies* against EBV *antigens*, notably the capsid antigen early in the disease and against EBNA (Epstein–Barr virus nuclear antigen) later, are usually present. Antibodies against *xenogeneic* red cells (notably horse and sheep) are also present and detected by the Paul–Bunnell *haemagglutination* test. See also *Burkitt's lymphoma* and *CR2*.

inflammatory cell Any cell present in an inflammatory lesion as part of the host response, e.g. *neutrophil leucocytes, eosinophil leucocytes, macrophages*, etc.

inhibition tests (1) Tests in which the activity of, e.g. a virus, is inhibited by the addition of dilutions of a *serum*, containing *antibody* which is being titrated. (2) Inhibition of a standard *agglutination, precipitation*, test, etc. by the addition of a purified preparation of the *antigen*, thus proving the specificity of the reaction. (3) See *hapten inhibition test*.

innate immunity See *native immunity*.

inoculation In immunology refers to introduction of a substance into the

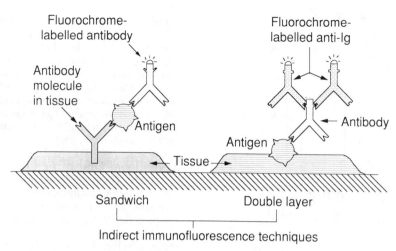

Figure I6. Indirect immunofluorescence techniques.

body, usually but not exclusively by *parenteral* (q.v.) injection.

iNOS (inducible nitric oxide synthase) See *nitric oxide*.

instructive hypotheses of antibody production Early hypotheses suggesting that *antibodies* have no specificity for *antigen* until they or the antibody-producing cells come into contact with it and therefore antigen instructs the cell to synthesize antibody specifically reactive against it; e.g. by acting as a template on which antibody is formed. Now replaced by *selective theories of the immune response.*

insulin dependent diabetes mellitus (IDDM; Type I diabetes mellitus) A form of diabetes especially frequent in young persons and due to autoimmune (see *autoimmunity*) destruction of insulin-secreting pancreatic islet beta cells. *Autoantibodies* and specific *T cells* against various islet cell *antigens* are detectable. These include cell surface antigens, the glucose transport protein and the enzyme glutamic acid decarboxylase. There is an association with HLA-DR3 and HLA-DR4 (see *HLA histocompatibility system*). Diabetics who carry these haplotypes have sequences in the DQ region which are different from those of DR3/DR4+ non-diabetics.

integrin superfamily A family of heterodimeric *Type I transmembrane proteins* each of which has an α and β chain. There are subfamilies determined by the β chain, thus β_1, β_2, etc., each of which may have multiple α chains. However, it is also clear that α chains can bind to more than one β chain, so the subfamily structure is not rigid. The β_2-integrins are also known as the leucocyte integrins (see *CD11/CD18*) since they are major mediators of *leucocyte* binding to vascular endothelium. This takes place in a first stage mediated by *selectins* (q.v.) which cause leucocytes to roll along the vessel wall, then a second stage in which integrins cause the leucocytes to stop, spread and transmigrate. Some of the β_1-integrins (VLA molecules, see *CD49*) are found on *lymphocytes* and perform the same function. Various other integrins have specific functions, e.g. $\alpha_4\beta_7$ is a homing receptor which allows lymphocytes to enter *Peyer's patches*. The cell surface *ICAMs* are *ligands* for integrins in leucocyte–endothelial interactions, but integrins also mediate binding of many cell types to extracellular matrix proteins such as fibronectin, laminin, vitronectin, etc. See also the table under *adhesion molecules*. See Table A2 and Figure I7.

interdigitating cell *Class II MHC antigen+* cell of *dendritic cell* mor-

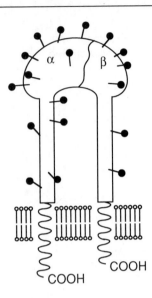

CD11a/CD18

Figure I7. Integrins. ⬤, N-linked glycosylation site.

phology found in the *T cell* areas of *lymph nodes* and other *lymphoid tissues*. Derived from *Langerhans cells* and other peripherally situated dendritic cells which, on contact with *antigen*, migrate up the afferent lymphatics to the lymph nodes. Important *accessory cells* because they present antigen (see *antigen presentation*) and provide the first contact site with antigen for recirculating *lymphocytes*.

interferons See *IFN-α, -β*; *IFN-γ*.

interleukin (IL) Definitions of the individual interleukins will be found under *IL-1, IL-2*, etc., which are the commonly used abbreviations. The name 'interleukin' is given to certain *cytokines* that act as intercellular signals. There is no logic to the interleukin designation: cytokines such as *IFN-γ* or *TNF-α* could as well be 'interleukins'. Nor is there any logic to the order in which the interleukins are numbered.

internal image Jerne's network theory postulates that, for every *antibody* against an external *antigen*, there is a set of antibodies of unrelated specificities bearing *idiotopes* that fit the *antigen-binding site* of the former antibody. These idiotopes will therefore have structures resembling that of the *epitope* on the external antigen and for this reason are said to constitute the internal image of the antigen. The production of antibody molecules with the properties of an internal image has been demonstrated experimentally in a small number of cases.

International Unit of Immunological Activity The potency of a given weight of an internationally accepted standard preparation of an immunological reagent (*antibody, cytokine*, etc.)

intraepithelial lymphocyte Any *lymphocyte* found within an epithelium particularly the intestinal epithelium.

intrinsic affinity Synonymous with *affinity* used in its strict sense, viz. to describe the interaction between a monovalent *hapten* and the *antigen-binding site* of the corresponding *antibody*.

intron A continuous sequence of DNA within a gene, flanked by *exons*, that does not code for amino acid sequences in the gene product. Many genes, including those for the *light chains* and *heavy chains* of *immunoglobulins*, contain introns. In *immunoglobulin genes*, introns separate the leader sequence (see *leader peptide*) from the *variable region*, the variable region from the *constant region* and the *hinge region* and homology regions of the heavy chain from each other. See Figure I4.

invariant chain (Ii; CD74) A trimeric intracellular protein which interacts on the *endoplasmic reticulum* with newly formed *class II MHC antigens* (α/β dimers) to form a complex which is incapable of binding peptide *antigens*. This means that, in the endoplasmic reticulum, which contains both class I and class II MHC antigens together with endogenously derived peptides, it is only the *class I MHC antigen* molecule that can bind these peptides. Ii also contains signal residues which target the class II α/β/Ii complex to an acidic and protease-rich endosomal compartment specialized for peptide loading, and in which the invariant chain is degraded. This compartment contains exogenously derived antigenic peptides of a size appropriate to bind to the invariant chain-free class II MHC α/β dimers in a form suitable for *antigen presentation*. See Figure A3.

Ir gene (immune response gene) Found within the *I region* (q.v.). Determines the capacity of an animal to mount an *immune response* against any defined *antigen*. See also *MHC genes*.

irradiation chimera Lethally irradiated animal whose *lymphoid tissues* and myeloid tissues have been successfully repopulated by haemopoietic cells transferred from another donor. Adult *bone marrow*, adult *spleen*, infant spleen and fetal liver have been shown to be effective repopulating tissues.

ISCOM (immune stimulating complex) Lipophilic particles formed by the spontaneous association of cholesterol, phospholipid and the saponin, Quil A®. Proteins incorporated into ISCOMs are highly *immunogenic* for all forms of *immune response* and the particles can be used as *vaccine* vectors. See also *liposome*.

isoantigen *Antigen* carried by an individual, which is capable of eliciting an *immune response* in genetically different individuals of the same species but not in the individual bearing it.

isoelectric focusing Technique for separating ampholytes (electrolytes, such as proteins and peptides, bearing both acidic and basic groups) according to their isoelectric point. A potential difference is applied across a system (liquid column, thin layer gel or cylindrical gel) in which pH increases from anode to cathode. Proteins or peptides present in the system focus into sharp bands in the region of the gradient corresponding to their own isoelectric point. Used widely in immunology; for instance *immunoglobulin* produced by a *B cell* clone focuses into a pattern of bands characteristic of that clone, the

clonotype or 'fingerprint' of the clone. See also *reverse immunoblotting*.

isogeneic (isogenic) Possessing absolutely identical genotypes, e.g. animals derived from the same egg, identical twins. Often used as a synonym for *syngeneic* as a descriptor of *inbred strains*. However, individuals of the latter are never absolutely identical in the sense implied by the term isogeneic. See also *transplantation terminology*.

isograft See *syngeneic* graft in Table T1.

isohaemagglutinin *Antibody* capable of reacting with *isoantigens* on the surface of erythrocytes and thus of *agglutinating* the cells. The naturally occurring antibodies against *ABO blood group system* antigens in human *serum* are examples of isohaemagglutinins.

isoimmunization *Immunization[1]* with *isoantigen*. Used in blood transfusion serology to refer to immunization of mother by fetal erythrocytes (see *erythroblastosis fetalis*) or recipient of a blood transfusion by donor erythrocytes of incompatible blood groups (see *incompatibility*).

isologous Sometimes used as a synonym for *isogeneic* or *syngeneic*, but note that these are subtly different.

isotype Classification of a molecule by comparison of its primary or *antigenic* structure with that of closely related molecules found within all members of the same species. Applied to the *immunoglobulins*, the isotype describes the *immunoglobulin class* and *immunoglobulin subclass*, *light chain* type and subtype and can also be applied to the *variable region* groups and subgroups. For example a mouse immunoglobulin may have isotype IgG_{2a} (κ) and its light chain may be from the variable region group V_κ-10. Cf. *allotype*, *idiotype*.

isotype switching A process that occurs during an *immune response* in which a *B cell* switches from production of one *immunoglobulin class* to another without loss of *specificity*. This is effected by the translocation of the VDJ *exon* from the *switch site* of the expressed *constant region* of the *heavy chain* to the switch site 5′ to the new heavy chain constant region. This process occurs in the order of the genes on the DNA, i.e. $\mu \rightarrow \gamma \rightarrow \varepsilon$ or α but cannot occur in reverse as the intervening DNA is excised and degraded. *Antibody* specificity is preserved since the heavy chain *variable region* sequence remains the same and there is no change in the *light chain*. Isotype switching is controlled by T_H2 *cell* cytokines such as *IL-4* and *IL-10*. There is evidence that, in some B cells, the VDJ exon is not translocated but a large mRNA transcript is produced, encompassing VDJ and some or all of the constant region exons. Different heavy chain isotypes are then produced by differential splicing of the mRNA. The δ chain (heavy chain of *IgD*) is always produced in this way as it has no switch site. See Figures I4 and I5.

isotypic variation Structural variability of *antigens* common to all members of the same species, e.g. the antigenic differences which distinguish the *immunoglobulin classes* and types of *immunoglobulin* chains. Cf. *allotype, idiotypic variation*.

ITP See *idiopathic thrombocytopenic purpura*.

J

J chain Polypeptide chain (MW 15 kD) with a high content of cysteine, found in the polymeric forms of *IgA* and *IgM*. Has been shown to link together two of the subunits in these *immunoglobulins* (see Figures I1 and I3), thus maintaining the polymeric structure. The J chains from IgA and IgM are identical and only one J chain is present in each molecule.

J exon (J [joining] gene) A short sequence of DNA coding for part of the third *hypervariable region* of the *light chain* or *heavy chain*, found near to the 5' end of the κ, λ and γ *constant region* exons but separated from them by an *intron*. Not to be confused with the *J chain* q.v. Several J exons are associated with each of the above constant region exons. In germ line DNA the *variable region* exon is separated from the J exon by a large region of untranslated DNA. During the differentiation of a *stem cell* to a *lymphocyte* a *V exon* is translocated to the position immediately 5' to one of the J exons to which it becomes attached.

J-gene See *J exon*.

Jennerian vaccination Jenner in 1798 described the use of infection with *cowpox* to induce *active immunity* in man that protected against smallpox (*variola*). His reputation rests on the fact that he proved the effectiveness of the method by *challenging*[2] the vaccinated boy James Phipps with virulent smallpox virus. His success was due to the fact that variola virus and cowpox virus share *cross reacting antigens*[2], yet the latter produces only localized lesions in man. It therefore stimulated protective immunity without causing serious disease. *Smallpox vaccination* as introduced by Jenner was still in use till recently but the vaccine virus, *vaccinia*, differed in some minor respects from the true cowpox virus.

Jerne plaque technique See *plaque-forming cell* (PFC) *assay*.

Job's syndrome See *hyper-IgE syndrome*.

Jones–Mote reaction Weak *delayed-type hypersensitivity* skin reaction seen on challenge a few days after *priming* with small amounts of protein *antigen* in aqueous solution or in *incomplete Freund's adjuvant* (not in *complete Freund's adjuvant*). A major feature is infiltration with *basophil leucocytes*. Possibly represents *T lymphocyte* mediated hypersensitivity modulated by *B lymphocytes*. Later challenge produces *Arthus reactions* or *weal and flare responses* q.v. See also *cutaneous basophil hypersensitivity*.

K

K cell (K [ADCC] cell; killer cell) Any cell which can exert a cytotoxic effect on target cells by using *antibody* to bind to them. Thus all cells with *Fc receptors* can bind to antibody-coated cells and *neutrophil leucocytes, eosinophil leucocytes, macrophages* and Fc receptor-positive *cytotoxic T lymphocytes*, may kill target cells following such binding. See *antibody-dependent cell-mediated cytotoxicity*.

kallikreins (kininogenases) Enzymes with indirect activity in increasing vascular permeability, vasodilatation and smooth muscle contraction. They are esterases which convert kininogens into pharmacologically active kinins q.v. Kallikrein activity is inhibited by *C1 inhibitor* q.v.

κ (kappa) **chain** One of the two types of *light chain* of *immunoglobulins*, the other being the **λ** (lambda) *chain*. An individual immunoglobulin molecule bears either two λ chains or two κ chains, never one of each. About 60% of human *IgG* molecules are of the κ type, 40% of the λ type but in the mouse the ratio is 95% to 5%.

K_d (dissociation constant) The reciprocal of the *association constant*. The dissociation constant is frequently quoted as a measure of the *affinity* of ligand–receptor (see *ligand* and *receptor*) interactions.

Kern An *antigenic* marker of human **λ** (lambda) *chains* resulting from the presence of glycine (Kern+) or serine (Kern–) at position 153. These are isotypic (see *isotype*) not allotypic (see *allotype*) markers. In combination with the *Oz* markers they define three isotypes of human λ chains.

keyhole limpet haemocyanin This substance, and haemocyanins obtained from other molluscs are excellent *antigens* in most vertebrates. Used as *carrier* in experiments designed to investigate the *immune response* to *haptens*.

killed vaccine See *inactivated vaccine*.

killer cell Term used for *K cells* q.v., and for a variety of other 'killer' cells, including *NK cells, cytotoxic T cells, neutrophil leucocytes* and *macrophages*.

kinins Peptides formed by the action of esterases known as *kallikreins* (kininogenases) and PF/dil on substrate kininogens present in plasma. Kinins have activity as vasodilators, increase vascular permeability and cause contraction of smooth muscle. One of them, *bradykinin* q.v., has been shown to be present in the blood during anaphylaxis.

KLH KLHC See *keyhole limpet haemocyanin*.

knockout mouse See *gene knockout mouse*.

Koch's phenomenon A phenomenon first observed by Robert Koch in 1891 when he inoculated living or dead *Mycobacterium tuberculosis* into guinea pigs that were already infected with the organism. A marked necrotic reaction occurred at the site, which sometimes became generalized and caused death. The same dead bacilli inoculated into healthy guinea pigs were innocuous. This reaction of *cell-mediated immunity* is the origin of the tuberculin test.

Kupffer cell A non-motile *macrophage* derived from blood *monocytes* and found lining the blood sinuses of the liver. As Kupffer cells are phagocytic (see *phagocytosis*) and positioned in an area of high blood flow they are highly active in removing foreign particles from the blood. In certain pathological conditions they also remove erythrocytes, the remains of whose haemoglobin forms golden-brown haemosiderin particles.

Kurloff cell Cell found in the peripheral blood, *spleen* and other organs of pregnant or oestrogen-treated guinea pigs. Contains a large inclusion body composed of mucoprotein and sulphated mucopolysaccharide and has been postulated to be a type of modified *lymphocyte* of unknown function.

L

L chain See *light chain*.

L-selectin (LECAM-1; MEL-14) See *selectins*.

LAK (lymphokine activated killer cells) *NK cells*, activated by *cytokines*, such as *IL-2*, that show an enhanced capacity to kill virus-infected cells or tumour cell targets.

λ (lambda) **chain** One of the two types of *light chain* of *immunoglobulins*, the other being the **κ** (kappa) *chain*. An individual immunoglobulin molecule bears either two κ chains or two λ chains, never one of each. The ratio of κ to λ chains varies with species, e.g. about 60% of human *IgG* molecules are of the κ type, 40% of the λ type, whereas in the mouse the ratio is 95% κ chains to 5% λ chains.

lamina propria Layer of connective tissue supporting the epithelium of the digestive tract and with it forming the mucosa. Contains the blood supply, lymphatic drainage and innervation of the mucosa and is the site of accumulation of *lymphocytes*, *plasma cells*, *mast cells* and *macrophages* in *immunological reactions* involving the gut.

Langerhans cell An *accessory cell* of dendritic appearance found in the basal layers of the epidermis, derived from *bone marrow* and characterized by the presence of tennis-racket shaped cytoplasmic Birbeck granules. Strongly *class II MHC antigen* positive, weakly positive for *Fcγ receptors* and *C3b receptors*. Weakly phagocytic (see *phagocytosis*). They are capable of processing and presenting protein *antigens* (see *antigen processing* and *antigen presentation*) but rapidly lose the capacity to process antigens on culture. However, cultured Langerhans cells have an enhanced capacity to present to class II MHC restricted *T cells* (see *MHC restriction*). Langerhans cells migrate from the skin to *lymph nodes* as immature forms of *dendritic cell*, q.v.

large granular lymphocyte A term describing the morphological appearance of *lymphocytes* found in human blood and tissue which are somewhat larger than *small lymphocytes* and in which cytoplasmic granules are prominent. Many have the phenotype and function of *NK cells* and the two terms are often used synonymously. However, *cytotoxic T lymphocytes* are also morphologically large granular lymphocytes.

late phase reaction Reaction which can begin about 5 hours after an *immediate hypersensitivity* reaction provoked by either *skin testing* or inhalation *challenge* by an *allergen*. The late phase reaction is characterized by inflammation, pruritus and a minimal cellular infiltration. The pulmonary form is thought to be closely related to chronic *asthma*; its mechanism probably due to late effects from the release of *cytokines* from *mast cells* or *alveolar macrophages*.

lattice hypothesis A hypothesis to explain the phenomenon that maximal *precipitation* is only seen at the point of *optimal proportions* when *antibody* and dilutions of soluble *antigen* are mixed. Postulates that *divalent* antibody molecules combine with the *epitopes* of *polyvalent* antigen molecules to form an insoluble macromolecular lattice at optimal proportions and soluble complexes in *antibody excess* and *antigen excess* (q.v.). First suggested by Marrack in 1934 and has received support from immunochemical and electron microscope studies of the antigen–antibody reaction.

lazy leucocyte syndrome Generic name for syndromes in children with recurrent infections, characterized by defective *neutrophil leucocyte* locomotion or *chemotaxis*. The term does not define any exact entity.

lck A T cell *protein tyrosine kinase* (member of the Src family) that noncovalently binds to the cytoplasmic domain of *CD4* or *CD8* and plays a role in *T cell* signal transduction.

LCM See *lymphocytic choriomeningitis*.

LD$_{50}$ The dose of toxin, or bacterial suspension, etc. that kills 50% of a test group of animals within a specified time. Used in the estimation of toxicity or virulence and for the measurement of the *challenge^2* doses of pathogenic organisms that are used in testing *vaccines*.

LE cell (lupus erythematosus cell) *Neutrophil leucocyte* containing *phagocytosed* nuclear material from other cells. Found in *SLE* in which bare cell nuclei may be *opsonized* by *anti nuclear antibody*. Formerly the basis of the 'LE test' which is now obsolete.

leader peptide (signal peptide) A sequence of approximately 20, mainly hydrophobic, amino acids found at the N-termini of most nascent secreted proteins, e.g. the *light chains* and *heavy chains* of *immunoglobulins*, but absent from the secreted form. The peptide is rapidly cleaved from the nascent chains once they are released into the *cisternal space* of the *endoplasmic reticulum* and is responsible for vectorial release of the polypeptide chains and hence their secretion from the cell: see *signal hypothesis*.

lectin Term originally restricted to proteins derived from plants that bind specifically to sugar groups including those of cell surface glycoproteins. Many of them are *mitogens* and have been widely used as *polyclonal activators* of *lymphocytes*, e.g. *concanavalin A*, phytohaemagglutinins (*PHA*). The term lectin is also used of many nonplant cell-membrane proteins that bind

carbohydrates and glycoproteins. Thus *CD23* and CD72 belong to a family of proteins called C-type lectins (C-type because carbohydrate-binding is calcium dependent). There is also a family of cell membrane 'S-type' lectins. *Selectins* are also carbohydrate-binding proteins.

leucocyte (leukocyte) The *white cells* of the blood and their precursors (see *myeloid cell series* and *lymphoid cell series*).

leucocyte adhesion deficiency (leucocyte adhesion defect; LAD) A serious form of *immunodeficiency* due to a defect in the β_2 integrin (see *integrin superfamily*) chain (*CD18*) which results in defective function of *leucocyte* integrins (*CD11*/CD18) and failure of leucocytes to adhere to, and transmigrate through, vascular endothelium. The major defect is in *neutrophil leucocyte* mobilization. The patients do not recruit neutrophils into sites of bacterial infection and do not form pus. The lesions tend to become necrotic. Patients have a neutrophil *leucocytosis* and the classical lesions of neutrophil function deficiency, i.e. severe infections of skin, lungs, etc. with pyogenic bacteria.

leucocyte common antigen Previous name for *CD45* q.v.

leucocytosis Increase above normal of the number of *leucocytes*, especially in blood.

leukocyte Alternative spelling of *leucocyte*.

leukotrienes Pharmacologically active substances generated from arachidonic acid by the action of lipoxygenases. They form a series of hydroxyeicosatetraenoic acids the most biologically active of which are:
   leukotriene B$_4$, (5, 12-dihydroxyeicosatetraenoic acid) which is chemotactic (see *chemotaxis*) for *neutrophil leucocytes* and other *leucocytes*;
   leukotriene C$_4$, (5-hydroxy-6-glutathionyl eicosatetraenoic acid);
   leukotriene D$_4$, a 6-sulphido-cysteinyl-glycine metabolite of leukotriene C$_4$;

leukotriene E$_4$, a 6-sulphido-cysteine metabolite of leukotriene D$_4$. Leukotrienes C$_4$, D$_4$ and E$_4$ together possess the activity of *slow reacting substance A* (SRS-A), i.e. they cause contraction of some types of smooth muscle, especially bronchial muscle, and they increase vascular permeability. Leukotrienes may be released from *mast cells, platelets* and various *leucocytes*, and SRS-A activity can be generated as a result of the combination of *antigen* with *IgE antibody*.

LFA-1 (CD11a/CD18) A *leucocyte* (β$_2$) integrin (see *integrin superfamily*) which binds to *ICAM-1, -2* and *-3* and is important for leucocyte endothelial attachment and for *lymphocyte–accessory cell* clustering. The *affinity* of lymphocyte LFA-1 for ICAM-1 increases transiently following activation, thus allowing attachment followed by detachment of cells. (LFA stands for leucocyte functional antigen which is now a meaningless term). See also *CD11* and Figures C3 and I7.

LFA-2 See *CD2*. The latter is the common usage.

LFA-3 (CD58) A member of the *Ig superfamily* that exists either as a *GPI anchor*-linked or as a *Type I transmembrane protein*. LFA-3 is found on most *leucocytes* and on endothelium. Strongly expressed on *macrophages*. It binds to *CD2* (LFA-2) which is a *T lymphocyte*-specific *antigen*. LFA-3–CD2 binding enhances T cell activation (see *lymphocyte activation*) and may be costimulatory. It also physically stabilizes clustering between T lymphocytes and *accessory cells*.

LGL See *large granular lymphocyte*.

ligand Something which binds. Term especially used of molecules which bind to cells or to other molecules.

light chain A polypeptide chain present in all *immunoglobulin* molecules. MW 22 kD in man. Immunoglobulins, or their subunits if polymeric, are made up of two identical light chains linked to two *heavy chains* usually by disulphide bonds (see Figure I2). Light chains are

of two *isotypes*, kappa and lambda (see κ (kappa) *chain* and λ (lambda) *chain*) and a single immunoglobulin molecule or subunit always has two κ chains or two λ chains, never both. Light chain isotype is not related to *immunoglobulin class* differences, i.e. all immunoglobulins of whichever class have κ or λ chains. Light chains have an N-terminal, *variable region* forming part of the *antigen-binding site* and a C-terminal, *constant region* which is invariable.

light chain subtype The subgroup into which a *light chain* is placed by virtue of features of its primary or *antigenic* structure, common to all individuals of the same species, which distinguish it from other light chains of the same type. As with *heavy chain subclass*, these structural features are found in the *constant region* but the differences between light chain subtypes are smaller than the differences between *light chain types*, e.g. human λ (lambda) *chain* subtypes are determined by the *Oz+, Oz–, Kern+* and Kern– antigenic markers. Three subtypes of mouse λ chains are known: λ$_1$, λ$_2$ and λ$_3$.

light chain type The group into which a *light chain* is placed by virtue of features of its primary or *antigenic* structure, common to all individuals of the same species, which distinguish it from other light chains. Only two light chains types have been found in all species examined to date, designated κ (kappa) *chain* and λ (lambda) *chain*.

light zone See *germinal centre*.

limiting dilution A technique of producing aliquots containing single cells (or microorganisms) by diluting a suspension to the point at which aliquots each contain a single cell. Effectively used to originate clones in e.g. *monoclonal antibody* production. May mislead unless additional tests are employed as, e.g. at the dilution at which, on average, one cell is present per aliquot, the cells will be distributed according to the Poissonian distribution to give 37% of aliquots with no cells and 63% with one or more than one cell each. Authentic clones can only be produced by methods that involve confirmation of the presence of a unique originating cell by visual or electronic means.

limiting dilution assay Any assay designed to quantify cells or microorganisms by diluting a suspension of them until aliquots on average contain single cells of the type being tested. In e.g. assays for *lymphocyte* precursors, the original suspension may contain an excess of other cells, the presence of which is required to enable detection of the assayed cell's activity. See also *limiting dilution*.

linkage disequilibrium The association of two or more *antigens* or genes in the same individual more frequently than would be expected by chance. Most commonly observed in the *HLA histocompatibility system*, e.g. HLA-A1, -B8 and -DR3 are found on the same chromosome more frequently than would be expected from the frequency of these alleles in the population.

lipocortin (annexin) Lipocortins are a series of anti-inflammatory proteins that are induced in cells by corticosteroids, and that are important mediators of the anti-inflammatory effects of corticosteroids. They act by preventing the release of inflammatory arachidonate metabolites (*prostaglandins* and *leukotrienes*). There are at least twelve related proteins with lipocortin activity. These proteins are called the annexin family.

lipopolysaccharide (LPS) Bacterial lipopolysaccharides are complex molecules consisting of a lipid core (lipid A) with a polysaccharide side chain. They are components of the O-antigen (*endotoxin* q.v.) complex of Gram negative bacilli especially enterobacteria such as *Escherichia coli*, *Salmonella* and *Shigella* spp. and also of *Haemophilus* and *Bordetella pertussis*. These all differ in antigenic structure, the difference in specificity being determined by differences in polysaccharide composition. Lipid A is incorporated into the outer membrane of the bacterium and the polysaccharide projects extracellularly. Lipid A is common to all lipopolysaccharides and mediates their physiological effects which are, therefore, similar whatever the organism. Bacterial lipopolysaccharides are characterized by their ability to produce *septic shock* with fall in blood pressure, increased adhesion of *leucocytes* to endothelium causing an initial leucopenia followed by a *leucocytosis*, pyrexia (hence called pyrogens) and general and local *Shwartzman reactions* q.v. Many of these effects are mediated by release of *cytokines* such as *IL-1* and *TNF-α*. They are also potent *adjuvants*, this activity being associated with lipid A, and are mitogenic (see *mitogen*) for murine *B lymphocytes*. They are often *thymus independent antigens* (*TI-1 antigens*).

liposome Spherical microstructure formed when mixtures of phospholipids with or without sterols are dispersed in aqueous solutions. Liposomes are made up of concentric phospholipid bilayers, and so form simple models of cell membranes which can be used for experimental studies. If *antigens* are incorporated in them, liposomes have been reported to act as *adjuvants*. See also *ISCOM*.

live vaccine *Vaccine* containing organisms that actively multiply or develop within the vaccinated host. Such vaccines often produce very strong and long lasting *protective immunity*. Strategies that have been, or are presently, widely used to prepare such vaccines include the use of: (a) attenuated strains of pathogens that are entirely non-pathogenic or cause acceptable reactions; (b) a different pathogen or attenuated strain of it that gives cross protection; and (c) the actual pathogen against which protection is desired. This is given either by an abnormal route, or at the same time as an *antiserum*, or, in the case of helminths, may be irradiated so that it is unable to complete development. See also *heterologous carrier vaccines*.

low dose tolerance *Immunological tolerance* in an immunologically mature animal induced by repeated very small doses of an *antigen*. Antigens that can be employed to induce tolerance some-times induce it in both high and low dose ranges but stimulate a normal *immunological response* at intermediate dose ranges. Cf. *high dose tolerance*.

low responder Term referring to *inbred strains* of laboratory animals which give poor *immune responses* to specified *antigens* when compared with other strains. Related to lack of *Ir genes* determining the response in question.

lpr^cg A mutation in the *fas* gene resulting in expression of *Fas* in a non-functional form. *Lymphocytes* of CBA/K1Jms mice, homozygous for *lpr^cg*, are defective in *apoptosis* and develop a lymphoproliferative disorder and, in female mice, an *autoimmune disease* resembling *SLE* (systemic lupus erythematosus), cf. *MRL-lpr/lpr mouse*.

LPS See *lipopolysaccharide*.

LPS binding protein A protein present at low levels in normal *serum*, but increased during an inflammatory response, that binds to the lipid A moiety of *lipopolysaccharide* (LPS). The LPS–LPS binding protein complex is then able to bind to *CD14* on the membrane of *mononuclear phagocytes* leading to activation of the functions of the latter.

LT (lymphotoxin; LT-α) LT is also known as *TNF-β* (q.v.). LT binds to another protein, named LT-β, which is found on the surfaces of cells on which it and LT (LT-α) form a complex that mediates the cellular effects of LT. Both LT and LT-β belong to the *TNF family* (q.v.).

lupus erythematosus Skin disease with red scaly patches in exposed areas especially butterfly-shaped area over the nose and cheeks. Not to be confused with lupus vulgaris, which is tuberculosis of the skin, nor with systemic lupus erythematosus (*SLE*, q.v.) of which cutaneous lupus erythematosus is often a sign and to which it is related.

lymph The fluid that flows past all tissue cells of the body thus providing a medium for metabolic exchange and

removal of waste products. Derived from the blood as an ultrafiltrate through the capillary walls it returns to the blood stream, after passing through chains of *lymph nodes* (q.v.), by drainage from the thoracic duct into the vena cava. It is similar in general composition to *plasma*; that draining the intestine and liver contains the most protein, fat in the form of chylomicrons is copiously present in mesenteric lymph. Most (80–85%) of the cells in normal lymph are *small lymphocytes*. Large *lymphocytes*, *monocytes* and *macrophages* are relatively rare except in lymph from areas of inflammation or sites of *immune responses*. A few erythrocytes and *eosinophil leucocytes* may normally be present. Afferent lymph (i.e. in lymphatics leading to lymph nodes) draining inflammatory sites may contain *inflammatory cells* and *accessory cells* such as macrophages and *veiled cells*. Recirculating lymphocytes (see *lymphocyte recirculation*) are found in efferent lymph (i.e. in lymphatics leading away from lymph nodes).

lymph node Small bean-shaped organ subdivided into a cortex and medulla and made up largely of *lymphocytes* and *accessory cells*, especially *dendritic cells* (*interdigitating cells*). The lymph node is a *peripheral lymphoid organ* and has both a lymphatic supply and a blood supply. The cortex is compartmentalized into *T cell* and *B cell* areas. Lymph nodes are distributed throughout the body, frequently in groups which drain *lymph* from a given area via afferent lymphatic vessels that pass into the node from peripheral tissue. An efferent lymphatic vessel passes from each lymph node to more central chains of nodes and, eventually, to the thoracic duct. The lymph nodes thus act as filters through which foreign materials including *antigens* must pass (often after being taken up by *accessory cells*) thus coming into contact with lymphocytes. Also *lymphocyte recirculation* of both T and B cells requires lymphocytes to enter the lymph node from the blood stream via *high endothelial venules*, to migrate to their respective (T and B) areas and eventually to leave via the efferent lymphatics. Lymph nodes are important centres for initiation and development of *immune responses*. Following antigenic *challenge*, responding B cells replace the *lymphoid follicles* to form *germinal centres*, and mature *antibody*-secreting *plasma cells* are found in the medulla. Likewise antigen-driven T cell maturation takes place in clusters around interdigitating cells in the *thymus dependent areas*. It should be noted that in some mammals, e.g. the pig, the classically described organization of the lymph node is reversed, the 'cortex' being close to the efferent lymphatic. See also *antigen processing* and *antigen presentation*. See Figure L1.

lymphoblast A *blast cell* (q.v.) of the *lymphoid cell series* with a nuclear pattern characterized by fine chromatin and basophilic nucleoli. Lymphoblasts are formed *in vivo* and *in vitro* following *antigenic* or *mitogenic* stimulation (see *lymphocyte activation*), and divide to form populations of *effector lymphocytes*. There are also many established lymphoblast lines widely available in long term culture. Many are *B cell* lines, fewer *T cell* lines.

lymphocyte The cell type that carries *receptors* for, and recognizes, *antigen* and is therefore the mediator cell of *specific immunity*. There are two major forms of mature lymphocyte, the *T lymphocyte* which generates the responses of *cell-mediated immunity*, and the *B lymphocyte*, which mediates *humoral immunity* and is the precursor of *antibody*-secreting cells. Unstimulated lymphocytes of both types are small cells (5–7 μm in diameter) with a large round or slightly indented nucleus and a narrow rim of cytoplasm. Following activation with antigen, the cells enlarge, proliferate, and differentiate into effector and *memory cells*. Lymphocytes are the major constituents of *lymphoid tissues* and are also found in peripheral tissues at sites where *immune responses* are taking place. Note that some cells of lymphocyte morphology (e.g. *NK cells*) lack receptors for antigen.

lymphocyte activation The change seen when *lymphocytes* are cultured in the presence of a *mitogen*, e.g. anti-*CD3* or *PHA*, or of an *antigen* to which they are *primed*. The cells enter the cell cycle sequence, typically remaining in G1 for about 48 hours before entering the S phase and dividing. They increase in size, the cytoplasm becomes more extensive, and nucleoli are visible in the nucleus, which becomes less densely stained; after about 72 hours these cells resemble *lymphoblasts*. Activated lymphocytes differentiate into various func-

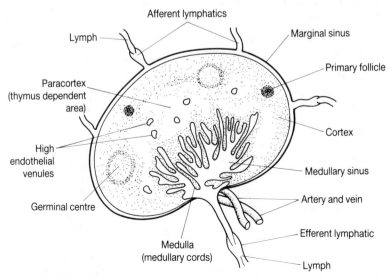

Figure L1. Lymph node.

tional forms, depending on the phenotype of the original cell, e.g. *B cells* to *memory cells* or *plasma cells, T cells* to *cytotoxic T lymphocytes, helper T lymphocytes, cytokine*-secreting cells, memory cells, etc.

lymphocyte recirculation The continuous passage of *lymphocytes* from blood to *lymphoid tissues* to *lymph* and thence back to blood. Recirculating cells are small resting cells which on passage through the *post-capillary venules (high endothelial venules,* HEV) of lymphoid tissues adhere specifically to, and migrate across, the high endothelial cells. They then traverse the lymphoid tissue by unknown mechanisms, eventually leaving via the efferent lymphatics from whence they reach major lymphatic channels and the thoracic duct which drains back into the bloodstream. Both *T cells* and *B cells* recirculate. There is tissue selectivity since, for example, mucosally derived lymphocytes recirculate back to mucosal lymphoid tissues. Once activated by *antigen*, lymphocytes lose selective affinity for HEV and leave the recirculating pool, migrating instead across non-specialized endothelium into sites of antigen deposition. See *homing receptors, addressins, selectins, GlyCAM-1* and *MAdCAM-1*.

lymphocyte transformation See *lymphocyte activation.*

lymphocytic choriomeningitis A viral disease of mice in which both the lesions and the capacity to clear the infection result from the generation of antiviral *immune responses* directed against virus infected cells. Infection may be acute or may progress to a persistent state. Persistent infection is due to a specific defect in the capacity to generate virus-specific, *MHC restricted, cytotoxic T lymphocytes.*

lymphocytosis Rise above normal of the number of *lymphocytes*, especially in blood.

lymphoid cell A *lymphocyte.*

lymphoid cell series Cell series which includes *lymphocytes*, their precursors,

e.g. *thymocytes,* and their progeny, e.g. *plasma cells*. Cf. *myeloid cell series.*

lymphoid follicle (primary follicle) A tightly packed, spherical aggregation of cells in the cortex of a *lymph node,* the white pulp of the *spleen* or in other *lymphoid tissues*. Consists of a network of *follicular dendritic cells,* the spaces between which are packed with small recirculating (see *lymphocyte recirculation*) mIgM+, mIgD+ (see *membrane immunoglobulin*) B *lymphocytes.* Lymphoid follicles characterize the B cell areas of unstimulated lymphoid tissue, but during the *secondary immune response* to *thymus dependent antigens, germinal centres* (q.v.) develop within the follicle (*secondary follicle*).

lymphoid tissues Body tissues in which the predominant cells are *lymphocytes.* They comprise the *lymph, spleen, lymph nodes, thymus, Peyer's patches,* pharyngeal *tonsils,* adenoids, and in birds the caecal tonsils (see *tonsils*) and *bursa of Fabricius.*

lymphokine Any *cytokine* made and secreted by *lymphocytes,* commonly following *antigen* stimulation, e.g. *IL-2, IL-4,* etc.

lymphoma Neoplastic disease of *lymphoid tissue* in which the abnormal cells are chiefly located in solid tissue, rather than found in the blood as in leukaemia, though there is overlap between the two. See *Hodgkin's disease, non-Hodgkin's lymphoma.*

lymphoreticular tissue Synonym for *lymphoid tissues.*

lymphotoxin (LT) Synonym for *TNF-β*.

lysin (1) *Antibody* which causes cell lysis, e.g. a *haemolysin*, or in *bacteriolysis*. (2) Other substances, especially bacterial toxins, which lyse cells.

lysosome A cytoplasmic organelle, limited by a membrane and containing hydrolytic enzymes (acid hydrolases). Present in many cells throughout the animals kingdom. Lysosomal enzymes are inert until released from the particle.

These enzymes play an important part in intracellular digestion and are involved in many types of cell injury. They may also be released from the cell by exocytosis. For role of lysosomes in *phagocytosis* see *phagosome*.

lysozyme Enzyme, first described by Fleming in 1922, present in and secreted by *neutrophil leucocytes* and *macro-phages* and found in tears, nasal secretions, on the skin, and, in lower concentrations, in *serum*. Lyses certain bacteria, chiefly Gram positive cocci. *Micrococcus lysodeikticus* is especially sensitive. A saccharolytic enzyme, it splits the muramic acid-β(1-4)-N-acetyl-glucosamine linkage in the cell walls of Gram positive bacteria. It also potentiates the action of *complement* on Gram negative bacteria (see also *IgA*).

M

M-CSF (macrophage colony stimulating factor; CSF-1) A homodimeric *cytokine* made by many cell types including *lymphocytes* and *activated macrophages*, that stimulates proliferation and differentiation of *monocyte* precursors to form mature monocytes. Thus more specific than *GM-CSF*. Also acts peripherally on differentiation of *macrophages*. Lack of its gene leads to deficiency of osteoclasts and to *osteopetrosis*. Also important for normal placentation and high levels are found in the uterus during pregnancy.

M-CSFR (macrophage colony stimulating factor receptor; CD115; CSF-1R) A *Type I transmembrane protein* of the *Ig superfamily* with four *constant regions* and one *variable region*, extracellular *immunoglobulin domains* and a cytoplasmic *protein tyrosine kinase* domain. Present on *mononuclear phagocytes* and their precursors and also in the placenta.

MAb (mAb) Abbreviation for *monoclonal antibody*.

MAC See *membrane attack complex*.

MAC-1 See *CD11*.

macroglobulin Any *globulin* with a molecular weight above about 400 kD. The best-studied *serum* macroglobulins are *IgM* (MW 970 kD) q.v. and α_2-macroglobulin (MW 820 kD). Many lipoproteins are also macroglobulins.

macroglobulinaemia Increase in level of *macroglobulin* in the *serum*. Usually refers to rise in *IgM* level. May follow *antigenic* challenge, e.g. in trypanosomiasis, or be due to *paraproteinaemia* either primary as in *Waldenström's macroglobulinaemia* or secondary to diseases such as *lymphoma* or carcinoma, especially in the alimentary tract.

macrophage The mature cell of the *mononuclear phagocyte* system q.v. Macrophages are derived from blood *monocytes* which migrate into the tissues and differentiate there. They are strongly phagocytic (see *phagocytosis*) of a wide variety of particulate materials, including microorganisms. They contain *lysosomes*, and possess microbicidal capacity. They are secretory cells which synthesize and release an enormous number of biologically active substances including *cytokines*, enzymes, inflammatory mediators, and microbicidal agents. Macrophages are strongly adherent to, and spread on, activated endothelia, and (*in vitro*) on protein-coated plastic or glass and show *chemotaxis*. They possess *Fc receptors* and *C3b receptors* and are *CD14+*. They stain positively for *non-specific esterase* and peroxidase. They can be divided into *class II MHC antigen*-negative and Class II-positive populations. The former are classical *phagocytes*, but the latter have an important role as *accessory cells* in *antigen processing* and *antigen presentation* to *lymphocytes* in induction of *immune responses*. See also *activated macrophage, elicited macrophage, resident macrophage*.

macrophage activating factor A generic term for any *cytokine* that activates *macrophages* (see *activated macrophage*), e.g. *IFN-γ, TNF-α, GM-CSF*.

MAdCAM-1 (mucosal addressin cell adhesion molecule) A *type I transmembrane protein* of the *Ig superfamily* found selectively on *high endothelial venules* of mucosal *lymphoid tissue* and in the lamina propria of the gut. It is an adhesion molecule which binds to the *lymphocyte* homing receptor $\alpha_4\beta_7$.

major histocompatibility complex (MHC) The collection of genes coding for the major *histocompatibility anti-gens*, see *class I MHC antigens, class II MHC antigens, HLA histocompatibility system* and *H-2 histocompatibility system*.

Malpighian body (Malpighian corpuscle) See *spleen*.

MALT Mucosa associated *lymphoid tissue*.

Mancini test See *single radial diffusion test*.

mannose-binding protein A protein of the collectin family (see *collectins*), found in normal human *plasma*, but absent or at low levels in a fairly common deficiency of *opsonization* in children with recurrent infections. Mannose-binding protein has direct opsonizing activity and also, when it binds to mannose-coated surfaces activates the *classical complement pathway*.

mantle zone (follicular mantle) A peripheral zone of small *B lymphocytes* found in a *secondary follicle* in which a *germinal centre* has developed. The mantle zone contains the small, recirculating, B cells which originally occupied the *primary follicle* but which have been pushed out as the germinal centre expands. See Figure G1.

Mantoux test An intradermal *tuberculin test* (q.v.) widely used in man. A positive test indicates *delayed-type hypersensitivity* to *Mycobacterium tuberculosis* and implies past or present infection with the bacillus. The test is negative during early stages of infection (about 3 weeks) and in rapidly progressing disease. After successful *BCG* vaccination a previously negative Mantoux test becomes positive.

marginal zone A loosely packed area of *T lymphocytes, B lymphocytes* and *macrophages* around the *periarterial lymphatic sheath* of the mammalian *spleen* q.v., particularly well-defined in rodents. Analogous areas are present in other *lymphoid tissues*. The marginal zone B cells are probably mainly B *mem-*

ory cells in G1 which, on *challenge* with *antigen*, migrate into the T cell areas (*thymus dependent areas*). See Figure S1.

margination Transient attachment of blood *leucocytes* to vascular endothelium. Normally, half of the *neutrophil leucocytes* in the blood are marginated at any given time. Margination also occurs at sites of inflammation where cells, which would normally not adhere, show a characteristic 'rolling' due to attachment by *selectins*. This is followed by a stronger integrin-mediated attachment (see *integrin superfamily*) and by migration out of the vessels.

mast cell Tissue cell (10–30 μm diameter) bearing high *affinity* surface *receptors* for *IgE* (FcεRI, see *Fcε receptors*) and strongly basophilic cytoplasmic granules, similar to, but smaller than, those of blood *basophil leucocytes*. The granules contain *histamine*, heparin, and tryptase, *inter alia*, and release of these and other, newly formed, pharmacological mediators, such as *prostaglandins, leukotrienes* (SRS-A), and *platelet activating factor* is mediated by *antigen* binding to mast cell-bound IgE antibody, or by *anaphylatoxins*. There are two phenotypically separate populations of mast cells. One, '*mucosal mast cells*' (q.v.), has sparse granules, a lymphoid appearance, is dependent on *T lymphocytes* for differentiation and is found in the gut in intestinal nematode infections. The other population, 'connective tissue mast cells', is richer in granules, T lymphocyte-independent, and present in *immediate hypersensitivity* and fibrotic lesions.

Masugi nephritis Experimental glomerulonephritis produced in one species (e.g. rat) by injection of *antibody* obtained from a second species (e.g. rabbit) that has been *immunized* with rat glomerular capillary basement membrane. If the dose of antibody is large, *glomerulonephritis* develops within 12 hours due to a reaction of the injected antibody with the (rat's) basement membrane followed by *complement* mediated tissue damage (see *immune complex disease*). With smaller doses of antibody, glomerulonephritis takes a few weeks to develop and results from an *immune response* to the foreign (rabbit) *IgG* which has become fixed to the basement membrane. Progressive chronic disease may follow from suitable dosing with antibody.

maternal immunity (maternally transferred immunity) *Passive immunity* (of *humoral immunity* type) acquired by the newborn animal from its mother. In man and other primates this is chiefly obtained before birth by the active transport of *immunoglobulins* across the placenta. The young of ungulates, in whom *antibody* is not transferred across the placenta, acquire it from the *colostrum* (q.v.) their intestines being permeable to immunoglobulins for a few days after birth. In all mammals *secretory IgA* in colostrum provides passive protection for the gut mucosa. The young of birds acquire maternal immunity from antibody in the egg yolk.

MCP See *membrane cofactor protein*.

MCP-1, -2, -3 *Monocyte* chemotactic (see *chemotaxis*) proteins (also known as MCAF, i.e. *macrophage* chemotactic and activating factor). Related β-*chemokines* with chemotactic and activating functions for *mononuclear phagocytes* but not for *neutrophil leucocytes* or *lymphocytes*. MCP-1 is an attractant for *basophil leucocytes*. MCP-3 attracts both basophil leucocytes and *eosinophil leucocytes*.

MDP See *muramyl dipeptide*.

medullary cord Area of the medulla of a *lymph node* close to the efferent lymphatic, composed largely of *macrophages* and, after antigenic stimulation, containing many *plasma cells*. See Figure L1.

medullary sinus Potential spaces in the medulla of a *lymph node* into which *lymph* drains before entering the efferent lymphatic. See Figure L1.

membrane attack complex Term used to denote the terminal *complement* components *C5*, *C6*, *C7*, *C8* and *C9*, which associate to form the terminal attack complex (C5b-9) on activation of either the *classical complement pathway* or the *alternative pathway*. C5b-9 contains a hydrophobic region which allows it to insert into lipid bilayers and cause cell lysis.

membrane cofactor protein (MCP; CD46) A *Type I transmembrane protein* of the *SCR superfamily* found on a wide variety of cells; *lymphocytes*, those of the *myeloid cell series*, *platelets*, endothelial cells, epithelial cells and fibroblasts. Acts as a cofactor to the enzyme *Factor I* to cleave *C3b* and *C4b*, restricting *complement* turnover.

membrane immunofluorescence An *immunofluorescence* technique using suspensions of living or paraformaldehyde-fixed cells so that when the *fluorochrome*-labelled reagent is applied it does not enter the cell and is only able to react with structures on the outer surface of the plasma membrane. Widely used to define cells phenotypically using a *fluorescence activated cell sorter* (FACS). Also used to study changes in topography of membrane components, e.g. clustering, *patching, capping*, etc. though this is best achieved by confocal microscopy.

membrane immunoglobulin (B lymphocyte receptor; mIg; sIg) *Immunoglobulin* on *B cells* in the form of a *Type I transmembrane protein*, thus synthesized by, and acting as the *antigen*-specific *receptor* of the B cell (see Figure C3). In *unprimed* cells, membrane immunoglobulin is of the *IgM* and *IgD* classes, but *isotype switching* (class switching) occurs during *T cell*-dependent *immune responses*, and these classes are replaced by IgG, IgA or IgE. Note that, since B cells have *Fc receptors*, immunoglobulin other than that produced by the cell itself may also be found on the cell surface.

memory cells *T lymphocytes* or *B lymphocytes* which mediate *immunological memory*.

metalophilic cells Cells which take up metal-containing stains, e.g. silver stains. This is a property of many cells of the *mononuclear phagocyte* system including the fixed *macrophages* of the *lymphoid tissues.*

methyl green pyronin stain A histological stain which colours DNA green and RNA red. It is useful for demonstrating cells whose cytoplasm contains large numbers of RNA-containing ribosomes, e.g. *plasma cells, lymphoblasts.*

MHC See *major histocompatibility complex.*

MHC genes (major histocompatibility complex genes) Genes that code for the cell membrane *major histocompatibility complex* antigens (HLA in man, H-2 in mouse, RT1 in rat). See *HLA histocompatibility system* and *H-2 histocompatibility system,* also *class I MHC antigens* and *class II MHC antigens.* See Figures H1 and H2.

MHC restriction The recognition by *T lymphocytes* of foreign *antigen* on the surface of a cell only in association with self-antigens of the *major histocompatibility complex. CD8+* T lymphocytes respond to foreign antigen in association with *class I MHC antigens,* whereas *CD4+* T lymphocytes respond to foreign antigen in association with *class II antigens.*

microfilaments Long, fine strands about 5–8 nm wide composed of helically polymerized actin and found, often as a network, in the cytoplasm of many eukaryotic cells including all immunological cells. Microfilaments are believed to mediate movement of the whole cell and of organelles within it. They form a contractile system which functions by the interaction of actin with actin-binding proteins and myosin. Cytoplasmic actin exists in equilibrium between a soluble and a polymerized form, so that microfilaments may undergo rapid assembly and disassembly as required by the cell. Microfilament function is probably essential in cell locomotion, *phagocytosis, phagosome–lysosome* fusion, exocytosis, cell division, etc.

microglobulin Any *globulin* or globulin fragment of relatively low molecular weight (40 kD or below). Has been used of low molecular weight proteins such as *Bence–Jones protein* in urine or similar proteins in *serum.* See β_2 *microglobulin.*

microphage Metchnikoff's term to describe *polymorphonuclear leucocytes* and other *phagocytic* cells of the *myeloid cell series* in contrast to *macrophages* q.v.

microtubules Long hollow cylindrical structures (tubular in cross section) with an outer diameter of about 20–25 nm, found in the cytoplasm of eukaryotic cells including all cells of the immune system. Composed chiefly of tubulin, a protein which exists in equilibrium between a soluble form and the polymerized tubular form, thus microtubules exist in equilibrium between assembly and disassembly. Kinesins (microtubule associated proteins) control the movement of organelles in the cytoplasm by allowing them to shuttle up and down the microtubule (from nucleus to plasma membrane and vice versa).

MIF See *migration inhibition factor.*

mIg See *membrane immunoglobulin.*

migration inhibition factor The first immunologically important *cytokine* to be described was a factor released in *delayed-type hypersensitivity* reactions, that inhibited *macrophages* from migrating out of capillary tubes. Still not unequivocally defined at the molecular level since several molecules with similar activities have been described.

minimal haemolytic dose (MHD) The lowest dose of *complement* capable of causing complete lysis of a set volume of a standard suspension of erythrocytes coated with anti-erythrocyte antibody (see *complement fixation test*).

minor lymphocyte stimulating antigen See *Mls.*

MIP-1α (macrophage inflammatory protein-α) A β-*chemokine* with chemotactic (see *chemotaxis*) activity for *mono-*

nuclear phagocytes, but not *neutrophil leucocytes*. Also has some attractant activity for *T cells, basophil leucocytes* and *eosinophil leucocytes*. Has important function as inhibitor of *stem cell* proliferation in the *bone marrow*.

MIP-1β (macrophage inflammatory protein-β) A *β-chemokine* with chemoattractant (see *chemotaxis*) activity for *mononuclear phagocytes* but not *neutrophil leucocytes*. May also be a *T lymphocyte* attractant.

mitogen Any agent which induces mitosis in cells. In immunology often used to refer to substances that are able to induce activation (see *lymphocyte activation*), DNA synthesis and cell division in a wide (polyclonal) range of *lymphocytes*.

mixed leucocyte reaction (MLR) *Lymphocyte activation* seen when mononuclear cells (mixtures of *lymphocytes* and *accessory cells*) from two genetically disparate individuals are cultured together *in vitro*. Due to a *cell-mediated immune* response of the cultured lymphocytes against foreign cell surface *antigens*. The strength of the reaction is directly related to the degree of *incompatibility* between the *histocompatibility antigens* of the two donors.

mixed lymphocyte reaction See *mixed leucocyte reaction*.

mixed vaccine (combined prophylactic) A *vaccine* containing *antigens* derived from several different species of pathogens, which gives protection against several diseases simultaneously. Cf. *polyvalent vaccine*.

MLR See *mixed leucocyte reaction*.

Mls (minor lymphocyte stimulating antigen) Antigens present on mouse *B cells* and possibly other *accessory cells* which stimulate a primary *mixed leucocyte reaction* (MLR) between cells from mice of identical *major histocompatibility complex* (MHC) *haplotypes*. Mls are protein products of ORF genes from endogenous retroviruses, such as mammary tumour viruses, which may integ-

rate with the genome. They are presented by *class II MHC antigens* and bind to the Vβ region of the *TCR* and they thus behave as self-*superantigens*.

modulation Disappearance of membrane proteins from the surface of a living cell after combination with their specific *ligands* or with specific *antibody*. Due to internalization of the complexed molecules.

monoclonal Pertaining to or derived from a single clone.

monoclonal antibody *Antibody* produced by a single clone of cells or a clonally derived cell line, and therefore having a unique amino acid sequence. Commonly used to describe the antibody secreted by a *hybridoma* cell line although strictly this is only monoclonal if one of the fusion partners is a nonproducer. Very widely used as a specific reagent for the identification and study of *antigens* and particularly useful when the latter have not been purified.

monocyte A large motile, amoeboid, phagocytic (see *phagocytosis*) cell with an indented nucleus. Found in normal blood (200–800 cells per mm^3 or 2–10% of the total *white cell* count in man). Derived from promonocytes in *bone marrow* and is the blood representative of the *mononuclear phagocyte* system. Monocytes remain in the blood for a short time (about 24 hours mean half-life) and then migrate into the tissues where they undergo further differentiation to become *macrophages*.

monokine Generic term for secreted products of *mononuclear phagocytes* with regulatory effects on their own functions or those of other cells, e.g. *IL-1, TNF-α*.

mononuclear cell A vague term often used to refer to cells of the *mononuclear phagocyte* system or to *lymphocytes* or to mixtures of the two as seen in histological sections or fractionated blood *leucocyte* samples; in contrast to *polymorphonuclear leucocytes*.

mononuclear phagocytes (mononuclear phagocyte system) A system of phagocytic cells of which the mature functioning form is the *macrophage*. The term mononuclear phagocyte system was introduced to replace the term 'reticuloendothelial system' which is now considered inaccurate. All mononuclear phagocytes are considered to share a common origin from the *bone marrow* promonocytes and to share a common function, i.e. *phagocytosis* and digestion of particulate material. If *class II MHC antigen*-positive they also act as *accessory cells*. A classification is given in Table M1 but it is probable that, under certain circumstances, macrophages of one type may take on the properties of another.

monospecific antiserum *Antiserum* against a single *antigen* or *epitope*. See also *monoclonal antibody*.

motheaten mouse A mouse with a defect of *T cell* and *B cell* maturation

associated with a recessive deficiency of a gene for a protein phosphatase.

MΦ (M phi) Abbreviation for *macrophage*.

MRL-*lpr/lpr* mouse An *inbred strain* of mouse *congenic* for the *lpr* (lymphoproliferative) gene. *lpr* has been identified with a defect in the *fas* gene causing diminished expression of *Fas*. *T cells* of MRL-*lpr/lpr* mice are defective in *apoptosis*, resulting in uncontrolled proliferation of double negative T cells (*CD4-*, *CD8-*) and enlargement of *lymph nodes*. Female mice of this strain develop an *autoimmune disease* resembling *SLE* (systemic lupus erythematosus). Other mouse strains congenic for *lpr* also exist.

MTT test (dimethylthiazol diphenyltetrazolium bromide) A yellow dye that is taken up in soluble form and converted

Table M1. Heterogeneity of the *mononuclear phagocyte* system

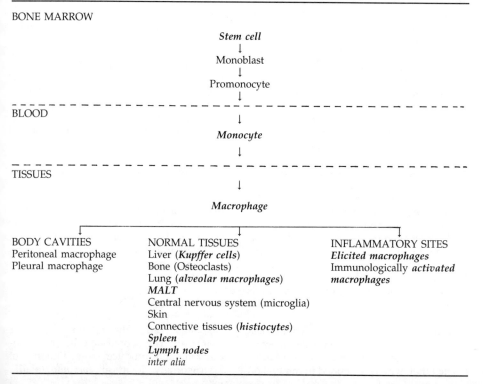

BONE MARROW

Stem cell
↓
Monoblast
↓
Promonocyte
↓
- -
BLOOD
↓
Monocyte
↓
- -
TISSUES
↓

Macrophage

BODY CAVITIES	NORMAL TISSUES	INFLAMMATORY SITES
Peritoneal macrophage	Liver (*Kupffer cells*)	*Elicited macrophages*
Pleural macrophage	Bone (Osteoclasts)	Immunologically *activated*
	Lung (*alveolar macrophages*)	*macrophages*
	MALT	
	Central nervous system (microglia)	
	Skin	
	Connective tissues (*histiocytes*)	
	Spleen	
	Lymph nodes	
	inter alia	

intracellularly to insoluble blue formazan only by living cells. Following cell lysis and solubilization of the formazan, it can be measured spectrophotometrically. A useful measure of cell viability. See also **nitroblue tetrazolium test**.

μ$_m$ (mu$_m$) The membrane form of the *heavy chain* of *IgM* (μ chain). See *membrane immunoglobulin* and also *tail peptide*.

μ$_s$ The secreted form of the *heavy chain* of *IgM* (μ chain) found in *serum*. Cf. **μ$_m$**.

mucosal mast cell Distinct population of *mast cells* found in mucosal tissues (especially intestine) characterized by production of specific serine protease and dependence on *T lymphocyte*-derived *IL-3* for growth.

multiple myeloma See *myelomatosis*.

multivalent vaccine See *polyvalent vaccine*.

muramyl dipeptide (MDP) N-acetyl-muramyl-L-alanyl-D-isoglutamine. The simplest structural unit of bacterial peptidoglycans capable of replacing the mycobacteria in *complete Freund's adjuvant* (q.v.) to produce *delayed-type hypersensitivity* and an elevated *antibody response* but reduced *granuloma* formation. It and its derivatives are weaker *adjuvants* than complete Freund's adjuvant and it has not found wide acceptance as an adjuvant for human use.

myasthenia gravis *Autoimmune disease* characterized by progressive muscular weakness on exercise caused by faulty neuromuscular transmission. The patients' *sera* contain *antibodies* against the acetylcholine receptor on the postsynaptic membrane of the neuromuscular junction. These antibodies are the putative cause of the symptoms and can induce autoimmune myasthenia gravis in experimental animals.

mycobacterial adjuvants Whole, heat killed, dried, mycobacteria (*M. tuberculosis, M. avium, M. phlei, M. smegmatis*, etc.) that, when suspended in mineral oil and emulsifier as in *complete Freund's adjuvant* have *adjuvant* activity in respect of any *antigen* given with them. The *immunological responses* to the antigen are greatly enhanced, especially that of *cell-mediated immunity*. They are commonly used to induce experimental *autoimmune diseases*, e.g. *experimental allergic encephalomyelitis* and, also, in the absence of added antigens, *adjuvant disease* q.v. Extracts of some mycobacteria, e.g. mycobacterial wax D and mycobacterial peptidoglycolipids have similar adjuvant activities. See also *muramyl dipeptide*.

myeloid cell series A series of *bone marrow*-derived cell lineages which include as mature forms the granular *leucocytes* (*granulocytes*) and the *mononuclear phagocytes* of blood. *Stem cells* become committed to the myeloid line under the influence of *GM-CSF* (see *colony stimulating factors*). *G-CSF* then causes maturation along the granulocyte line into myeloblasts then to myelocytes which, in turn, mature into granulocytes (*neutrophil leucocytes*). Alternatively *M-CSF* (CSF-1) causes maturation along the mononuclear phagocyte maturation pathway to *monocytes*. Mature neutrophils and monocytes are released into the circulation and are present in normal blood. This maturation process is known as myelopoiesis. *Eosinophil leucocytes* and *basophil leucocytes*, though related, follow different pathways of development from neutrophils and monocytes. See also *lymphoid cell series*.

myeloma A tumour of *plasma cells*, see *plasmacytoma, myelomatosis*.

myeloma protein *Immunoglobulin* that is *monoclonal* produced by neoplastic *plasma cells* in *myelomatosis* in man, mouse and other species. Detected as an electrophoretically homogeneous *paraprotein*.

myelomatosis Disease characterized, in man, by neoplastic proliferation of *plasma cells* throughout the *bone marrow*. The neoplastic cells are *monoclonal* and produce large amounts of structurally identical *immunoglobulin* (*paraprotein*) usually of *IgG* or of *IgA* class though *IgD* and *IgE* have also been reported, forming a sharply localized band on *serum* electrophoresis and a characteristic monoclonal banding pattern on *isoelectric focusing*. *Bence–Jones protein* appears in the urine in a proportion of cases. Myelomatosis may present with anaemia due to bone marrow replacement or with spontaneous fractures of bone. Commonest in men over 50 years and usually fatal. See also *plasmacytoma* and *paraproteinaemia*.

myeloperoxidase Peroxidase found in the *azurophil granules* of the *neutrophil leucocyte*, which, together with hydrogen peroxidase and halide, forms a bactericidal system. Families with myeloperoxidase deficiency have been reported.

N

naive lymphocyte A *lymphocyte* that has not met *antigen*. An *unprimed* lymphocyte.

NAP-2 See Table C2.

native immunity *Non-specific immunity* resulting from the genetic constitution of the host, e.g. *immunity* of man to canine distemper.

natural antibody *Antibody* present in *serum* of normal individuals not known to have been immunized (see *immunization*) against the relevant antigen. Examples in man include the *isohaemagglutinins* of the *ABO blood group system* and antibodies to the *Forssman antigen*. They possibly result from an immune reaction against some closely related antigen, e.g. blood group antibodies may be directed against closely related antigens of bacteria or food in the intestine of the infant.

natural fluorescence See *autofluorescence*.

natural immunity See *native immunity*.

natural killer cell See *NK cell*.

naturally acquired immunity *Immunity* acquired by random exposure to *antigen* as opposed to immunity acquired as a result of deliberate *immunization*.

NBT See *nitroblue tetrazolium test*.

negative phase A drop in antibody *titre* seen immediately after the administration of a second or later dose of *antigen* to a *primed* animal. Due to combination of the antigen with pre-existing *antibody* in the circulation.

negative selection *Clonal deletion* of *antigen*-specific, *receptor* bearing, *lymphocytes*, resulting in permanent loss of the relevant cells and their progeny. Term usually applied to the deletion of self (*autoantigen*)-reactive *T lymphocytes* during development in the *thymus*, but may also refer to elimination of self-reactive *B lymphocytes*.

neoantigen An *antigen* detected in the body during a disease state which is not found in health. Does not apply to the commonly recognized antigens of pathogenic organisms. Term used particularly in tumour studies, when a tumour antigen is found which is not detected in normal fetal or adult tissues.

neonatal thymectomy syndrome See *wasting disease*.

network theory A theory proposed by N. K. Jerne that the immune system is controlled by a network of interacting *antigen-binding sites* (paratopes) and idiotypic determinants (*idiotopes*) on *immunoglobulin* molecules and *lymphocyte* antigen *receptors*. Each paratope is capable of recognizing an *epitope* on an external *antigen* and also an idiotope on another immunoglobulin molecule (the '*internal image*'). Since each immunoglobulin molecule bears an idiotope, for which there is a corresponding paratope, this results in a network of interactions. It is postulated that interaction between two components of the system can result in stimulation or suppression, depending upon the nature of the interaction, the end result being a balanced system. This system is disturbed by the introduction of an external epitope, until a new dynamic equilibrium is reached. Although components of the system (idiotope, anti idiotope, internal image) have been observed, it has never been conclusively demonstrated that the immune system as a whole operates in the manner described by this theory.

neutralization test Any test in which *antibody* is measured by its capacity to neutralize the biological effects produced by an *antigen* or by an organism bearing it, e.g. neutralization of the infectivity of a virus or the biological effects of a bacterial toxin. See *phage neutralization test, virus neutralization tests*.

neutrophil leucocyte Cell of *myeloid cell series*, the most numerous in normal peripheral blood (normal count in human blood 2500–7500 per mm^3 or 40–75% of the total *white cell* count.). A motile, short-lived cell with multilobed nucleus and a cytoplasm filled with *azurophil granules* q.v. and *specific granules* q.v. which do not take up acidic or basic dyes strongly (hence name). Actively phagocytic (see *phagocytosis*) with an efficient microbicidal capacity (see *reactive oxygen intermediate*). Also reacts vigorously to chemotactic stimuli (see *chemotaxis*). The major cell in acute inflammatory lesions, e.g. acute bacterial infections, also *Arthus reactions*. Name usually abbreviated to neutrophil. Also known as polymorph or polymorphonuclear leucocyte or granulocyte (*eosinophil leucocytes* and *basophil leucocytes* also have multilobed nuclei and cytoplasmic granules). It should be noted that in species other than man, the blood cells acting functionally as neutrophils may have granules whose staining properties are not 'neutrophil'. These are sometimes known as heterophil granulocytes.

New Zealand black mouse See *NZB mouse* also *NZW mouse* (New Zealand white mouse).

NF-AT (nuclear factor of activated T cells) A protein complex which binds to DNA and is essential for transcription of the genes for *IL-2*, and other *cytokines* in *T cells*. Its activity is regulated by *calcineurin* phosphatase and thus inhibited by *cyclosporin A* and *FK506*®.

NGFR superfamily (nerve growth factor receptor superfamily) See *TNFR superfamily*.

nitric oxide (NO) A highly reactive, colourless and odourless gas. In biological systems it has a half-life between 3 and 15 seconds and is derived from molecular oxygen and the guanidino nitrogen of L-arginine, in a reaction catalysed by NO synthase (NOS). Certain cells, e.g. vascular endothelium, generate NO through a constitutive NOS (cNOS, calcium-dependent). This mediates vascular relaxation. Functions such as neurotransmission and *platelet* aggregation are mediated through a similar constitutive pathway. Another form of NOS is inducible (iNOS, calcium-independent) by immunological stimuli such as *IFN-γ, TNF-α* and *lipopolysaccharide* to produce large amounts of NO which can be cytotoxic. This is an important microbicidal function of *activated macrophages*.

nitroblue tetrazolium test Test of *neutrophil leucocyte* function. Nitroblue tetrazolium is a soluble yellow dye which is taken up into neutrophils only when they are exposed to a phagocytic (see *phagocytosis*) stimulus. Normal neutrophil NADPH oxidase reduces the dye which is then deposited as insoluble deep-blue formazan crystals within the cell. Neutrophils from patients with *chronic granulomatous disease* q.v. lack the capacity to reduce nitroblue tetrazolium. See also *MTT test*.

NK cell (natural killer cell) Cytotoxic *lymphocytes* which lack the phenotypic markers of both *T cells* (*TCR, CD3*) and *B cells* (*membrane immunoglobulin*). Normally present as a minority population in blood. They contain prominent cytoplasmic granules and are morphologically distinguishable as *large granular lymphocytes*. They bear FcγRIII (CD16, see *Fcγ receptors*) and *CD56* as characteristic markers. They are able to kill virally infected cells and certain sensitive tumour cells, though the mechanism by which they recognize these cells is not understood. It is not *antigen*-specific or *MHC restricted*, but the mechanism of killing is similar to that of *cytotoxic T lymphocytes*. NK cell granules contain *granzymes* and the cells release *perforins* which are inserted into the membrane of the target cell. Activated

NK cells also make *IFN-γ* and other cytokines. NK cell activity does not require prior stimulation, but is enhanced by the action of *cytokines*, e.g. *IL-2*. Cytokine-activated NK cells are known as *LAK* cells.

NK cell stimulating factor See *IL-12*.

NKSF See *IL-12*.

NO See *nitric oxide*.

NOD mouse See *non-obese diabetic mouse*.

non-Hodgkin's lymphoma A group of neoplastic diseases of *lymphoid tissue*, in most of which the abnormal cells are *B cells* and are usually derived from *germinal centre* cells. They vary from small lymphocytic *lymphomas* consisting of *CD5+* B cells, which resemble *chronic lymphocytic leukaemia* B cells and are of low malignancy, to high-grade-malignancy *centroblastic* lymphomas. Histologically the lymphomas may be follicular or diffuse. There are many variants whose classification is complex. The definition includes *Burkitt's lymphoma*.

non-identity, reaction of See *reaction of non-identity*.

non-immune animal Animal which has not been *primed* with a given *antigen*.

non-obese diabetic mouse *Inbred strain* of mouse that spontaneously develops insulin-dependent diabetes mellitus, due to *autoimmune* destruction of the islets of Langerhans cells in the pancreas.

non-specific esterase (alpha-naphthyl acetate esterase) Enzyme identifiable within *mononuclear phagocytes* and some *lymphocytes* by cytochemical staining. Mononuclear phagocytes show characteristic diffuse, granular cytoplasmic staining and this is commonly used as a criterion for identifying these cells. A proportion of human *T lymphocytes* also stains for non-specific esterase, but

with a quite different appearance of a single, or small number of localized, discrete dots.

non-specific fluorescence In *immunofluorescence* tests, fluorescence emitted for reasons unrelated to the specific combination between *antibody* and *antigen*. May be due to the presence of free *fluorochrome* or to fluorochrome labelling of proteins other than the antibody under test (especially *albumin*, α, β *globulins* in *serum* or unwanted antibodies). See also *autofluorescence*.

non-specific immunity Mechanisms for the disposal of foreign and potentially harmful macromolecules, microorganisms or metazoa which do not involve the recognition of *antigen* and the mounting of a specific *immune response*. Such mechanisms include the action of *lysozyme* or anti-viral *interferons*, *phagocytosis* and chemical and physical barriers to infection. *Protective immunity* in invertebrates is of the non-specific type. Specific and non-specific immunity are so closely linked in vertebrates that it is often impossible to dissociate their actions, cf. *specific immunity*.

non-tissue specific antigen *Antigen* present in more than one normal tissue or organ, e.g. nucleoprotein. Cf. *tissue specific antigen*.

northern blotting A technique for the detection of RNA molecules containing defined sequences. RNA molecules of different sizes are separated into bands by electrophoresis in Agarose® gel and transferred to a membrane by capillary blotting, which produces an exact replica of the original pattern on the membrane. Bands of RNA containing defined sequences, e.g. specific mRNA, are detected by hybridization with radiolabelled cDNA. Widely used in molecular immunology. See also *Southern blotting*.

NOS (nitric oxide synthase) See *nitric oxide*.

nu nu **mice** See *nude mice*.

nude mice Mice with congenital absence of the *thymus*, and whose blood and *thymus dependent areas* of the *lymph nodes* and *spleen* are depleted of *T lymphocytes*. These mice are homozygous for the gene 'nude', abbreviation *nu*, hence *nu nu*, and have no hair. They should be distinguished from mice carrying other genes that cause a lack of hair, e.g. shaven *Sha*; hairless, *hr*; bare, *ba*; hair loss, *hl*; etc. All these latter strains have normal thymuses. See also *thymic hypoplasia*.

null lymphocyte A *lymphocyte* that has no detectable *membrane immunoglobulin* (mIg), or *T lymphocyte* markers (*TCR, CD3, CD2*) on its surface, cf. T lymphocyte and *B lymphocyte*. *NK cells* are null lymphocytes.

nurse cell See *thymic nurse cell*.

NZB mouse (New Zealand black mouse) *Inbred strain* of mouse which develops spontaneous *autoimmune* haemolytic anaemia. They show a positive *antiglobulin test* between 4 and 10 months of age, at which time glomerular and tubular renal lesions (and extra-medullary haemopoiesis) are also seen. There is some evidence that this *autoimmune disease* may be of viral aetiology. See also *NZW mouse*.

NZW mouse (New Zealand white mouse) An *inbred strain* of mouse. Although immunologically normal, females of the F_1 *hybrid* between *NZB mice* and NZW mice develop an *autoimmune disease* resembling *SLE* (systemic lupus erythematosus).

O

oligosaccharide determinant A small number (2–7) of 5, 6 or 7 carbon sugars (pentoses, hexoses or heptoses) joined by glycoside linkages, that form the *epitope* on a polysaccharide *hapten*.

opsonin Factor present in plasma and other body fluids which binds to particles, especially cells and microorganisms, and increases their susceptibility to *phagocytosis*. Opsonins may be: (a) *Antibodies* which bind to *epitopes* on the particle. Particle-bound antibody can then attach by its *Fc fragment* to the *Fc receptors* of *phagocytes* thus initiating phagocytosis of the particle. (b) Products of *complement activation* esp. *C3b*. These are known as heat-labile opsonins. (c) Other non-antibody, non-*complement* opsonins (e.g. fibronectin) have also been found in biological fluids. See *mannose-binding protein*.

opsonization Coating of microorganisms and other particles with *opsonins* thus facilitating their *phagocytosis*.

optimal proportions In *precipitin tests*, if *antibody* and *antigen* are present in such a ratio that the maximum combination between *antigen-binding sites* and *epitopes* can occur, they are said to be present in optimal proportions or 'at equivalence'. At this ratio, maximum *precipitation* occurs. Cf. *antibody excess*, *antigen excess*, and see *lattice hypothesis*.

oral tolerance The induction of specific *immunological tolerance* by oral administration of *antigen*. This is the usual result of feeding soluble antigens (e.g. food proteins) to a naive animal (*non-immune animal*).

organ specific antigen See *tissue specific antigen*.

original antigenic sin Term first used to describe a phenomenon in which, after *vaccination* or infection with influenza virus, followed by re-infection or vaccination with a related but not identical virus, the *antibody* produced in response to the second virus is still directed against the first virus. Also used in more general contexts to describe similar phenomena.

orthotopic graft Tissue or organ grafted to a site normally occupied by that tissue or organ. Cf. *heterotopic graft*.

osteopetrosis 'marble bone disease'. Due to deficiency of osteoclasts normal resorption and remodelling of bone does not take place. The bone becomes brittle and liable to fracture. Osteoclasts are *mononuclear phagocytes* and the disease is associated with a genetic deficiency of *M-CSF*. It has been corrected in osteopetrotic (op/op) mice by *transfection* of the CSF-1 gene. Osteopetrosis is also associated with a generalized deficiency of macrophages, poor growth and a short life span.

Ouchterlony test *Precipitin test* of *double diffusion test* type. Wells are cut in a plain agar plate and filled with appropriate solutions of *antigen* and *antibody* which then diffuse through the agar gel and meet to form lines of precipitate (see *precipitation*). See *reaction of identity*, *reaction of partial identity*, *reaction of non-identity* and *spur*.

ovalbumin (OA; OVA) A negatively charged protein obtained from the white (albumen) of the avian egg. Unrelated to the *albumin* of fowl serum. Frequently used as an experimental *antigen*.

oxazolone (4-ethoxymethylene-2-phenyl-oxazol-5-one) A chemical employed to produce experimental *contact hypersensitivity*.

oxidative metabolic burst (respiratory burst) The rapid generation of *reactive* oxygen intermediates (q.v.) in neutrophil leucocytes and mononuclear phagocytes following phagocytosis and related stimuli (e.g. chemotactic factors).

Oz Oz+ and Oz– are antigenic markers on human λ chains defining λ subtypes.

Oz+ λ chains have lysine at position 191 whereas Oz– chains have arginine at the same position. In combination with the Kern markers (q.v.) they define three human λ chain subtypes.

P

P Symbol for *properdin*.

P-selectin See *selectins*.

PAF See *platelet activating factor*.

PAGE See *polyacrylamide gel electrophoresis*.

PALS See *periarteriolar lymphatic sheath*.

panning Method for purifying cells from a mixture by coating a surface such as a dish with an *antibody* specific for one of the cell types in the mixture. These cells will adhere to the surface and the non-adherent cells can be removed. For example, *CD4*+ and *CD8*+ *T cells* can be separated in this way.

PAP technique See *peroxidase–anti peroxidase technique*.

papain hydrolysis The reaction by means of which *IgG* molecules are split into three fragments (two *Fab fragments* and one *Fc fragment*) by treatment with papain (a protease derived from the papaw plant *Carica papaya*) in the presence of cysteine. Papain attacks a histidyl-threonine peptide bond in the *hinge region* of the *heavy chain* as shown in Figure I2.

paracortex The *thymus dependent area* of a *lymph node*.

paraprotein Any abnormal protein in *serum* but usually refers to *immunoglobulin* derived from an abnormally proliferating clone of neoplastic *plasma cells*. Paraproteins are normally *monoclonal* and appear as a sharply localized band on serum electrophoresis. *Myeloma proteins* and the abnormal *IgM* of *Waldenström's macroglobulinaemia* are examples of paraproteins.

paraproteinaemia Presence in *serum* of *paraprotein*. A diagnostic feature of *myelomatosis* and *Waldenström's macroglobulinaemia*. (See also *benign monoclonal gammopathy* and *α chain disease*.) Paraproteinaemias involving all five *immunoglobulin classes* have been reported in man, the frequency in any given class being proportional to the normal serum concentration of that class. Also occurs in mice, see *plasmacytoma*.

paratope Synonym for *antigen-binding site*.

parenteral Introduced or injected into the body by any route other than through the alimentary canal.

paroxysmal cold haemoglobinuria Disease in which haemoglobin appears in urine following exposure to cold. Due to presence in *serum* of *Donath–Landsteiner antibody* which binds to erythrocytes in the cold and lyses them on warming in the presence of *complement*.

paroxysmal nocturnal haemoglobinuria (PNH) A rare disease in which red cell membranes are abnormally sensitive to *complement*-mediated lysis. There is a defect in the synthesis of the *GPI anchor* and, in consequence, defective insertion of GPI-anchored proteins into cell membranes. Thus the disease affects not only erythrocytes but other *bone marrow*-derived cells and there may be defects of *leucocytes*, e.g. *neutrophil leucocytes*. The erythrocytes lack *decay accelerating factor* and also *CD59* (protectin), the latter defect causing the erythrocytes to activate complement directly and hence to lyse (see *PNH cells*).

partial identity, reaction of See *reaction of partial identity*.

particulate antigen An insoluble particle such as a cell or bacterium or fragments of these, carrying *antigens*, usually numerous with diverse *epitopes*. Alternatively an inert insoluble particle (or cell, or large fragment thereof, etc.) to which soluble antigens are adsorbed (see *adsorption*). *Antibodies* against particulate antigens can be demonstrated by *agglutination tests* and are often of the *IgM* class.

passive agglutination test A test used to detect antibodies to soluble *antigens*. Molecules of the latter are firmly attached to small particles of uniform size such as polystyrene latex, or erythrocytes. *Agglutination* of these passive supports occurs when *antibody* to the antigen is present. See *tanned red cell test*.

passive Arthus reaction Artificially induced skin lesions of *Arthus reaction* type produced by passively administering large quantities of precipitating *antibody* (see *precipitation*) by the intravenous route, and then inoculating the corresponding *antigen* subcutaneously or intradermally. In contrast to *passive cutaneous anaphylaxis* (q.v.) the antibody need not have been produced in the same species of animal as that in which the test is carried out.

passive cutaneous anaphylaxis *In vivo passive transfer* technique for recognizing and quantifying *IgE* antibody responsible for *immediate hypersensitivity* reactions. An animal is injected intradermally with *antibody* from the same species and a sufficient interval is allowed for fixation to cells of any IgE present and diffusion away of non-cell-fixed antibody. *Antigen* is then injected intravenously mixed with the dye Evans blue. Where the antigen reacts with cell-fixed antibody *vascular permeability factors* are released, the permeability of the vessel walls increases and *plasma* and the dye leak out giving a blue spot on the skin the size of which can be measured.

passive haemolysis Erythrocyte destruction following the binding of *antibody* to an erythrocyte surface *antigen* in the presence of *complement*. The antigen need not be a membrane protein but may be an antigen *adsorbed* or deliberately attached to the red cell surface.

passive immunity *Immunity* due, not to the production of a specific *immune response* by an individual, but to the presence in their tissues of *antibody* or *primed lymphocytes* derived from another *immune* individual. Examples are the immunity of the neonate against many infectious agents due to placentally or colostrally transferred maternal antibody (see *maternal immunity*) and the use of *antitoxins* to give protection against diphtheria or tetanus. In the case where lymphocytes are transferred (*adoptive transfer*), the term *adoptive immunity* is often used.

passive immunization The use of *antibody* or *primed lymphocytes* from an *immune* individual to produce *passive immunity* against an *antigenic* substance (e.g. toxin) or organism in a *non-immune animal* or individual. Gives short-lived *immunity* so its use is restricted to therapy or short-term prophylaxis and it is not suitable for long-term protection, cf. *active immunization*. Examples in man: use of *diphtheria antitoxin* to treat the disease; tetanus antitoxin as a precaution with deep, contaminated, wounds; and *gamma globulin* in *antibody deficiency syndromes*. Amongst numerous applications in animals the passive immunization of newborn lambs against clostridial diseases may especially be noted. This is accomplished by strategic *vaccination* of ewes before lambing so that their *colostrum* contains large amounts of antibody at that time. See also *maternal immunity*.

passive sensitization *Passive transfer* of *hypersensitivity* from a *primed* donor to a normal host by administration of *antibody* or *primed lymphocytes*. See also *passive cutaneous anaphylaxis*, *adoptive transfer*.

passive transfer Transfer of *immunity* or *hypersensitivity* from an *immune* or *primed* donor to a previously *non-*

immune animal by injection either of *antibody* or *primed lymphocytes*.

patch tests Tests used in the diagnosis of skin allergies (see *allergy*) particularly those of the *contact hypersensitivity* type, e.g. to nickel. The suspected substance is applied to the skin for a short period under an impervious dressing. A positive result is one that reproduces the original allergic condition.

patching Appearance of cell surface observed using *membrane immunofluorescence* or other labelling techniques after a polyvalent *ligand*, e.g. *antibody*, has been allowed to react with surface molecules on a cell membrane. Cross-linking of the molecules by the ligand causes them to form clusters which resemble a two-dimensional *agglutination* reaction. Occurs because membrane components are able to diffuse laterally in the plane of the membrane producing a patchy surface fluorescence. Does not require metabolic energy on the part of the cell and can be demonstrated at 4°C, cf. *capping*.

PCA See *passive cutaneous anaphylaxis*.

PCR See *polymerase chain reaction*.

PECAM See *CD31*.

penicillin hypersensitivity *Hypersensitivity* to breakdown products of penicillin such as penicilloic or penicillenic acid acting as *haptens* and binding to the patient's own proteins. Often manifested as a drug rash or as *serum sickness* with fever, joint pains and urticaria following orally administered penicillin, but *parenteral* administration can result in *anaphylaxis* (rare).

pentraxin A group of related proteins with a pentameric organization of identical subunits found in normal *plasma*, and at increased levels during inflammatory responses, hence they are *acute phase reactants*. The family includes *C reactive protein* and serum amyloid P component, see *amyloidosis*.

pepsin digestion Use of the gastric enzyme pepsin to split the polypeptide chains of proteins. It attacks certain peptide links between L-dicarboxylic and L-aromatic amino acids. In immunology, its chief use is to split *immunoglobulin* molecules in the *hinge region* giving a *F(ab')₂ fragment* q.v. plus small peptide fragments derived from the *Fc fragment*, see Figure I2. This has a practical use inasmuch as the *IgG* molecules of *antitoxins* used in *passive immunization* can be treated with pepsin and the F(ab')₂ fragments separated (termed *despecification*). These fragments retain their activity as divalent *antibody* but, on injection, are less likely to give rise to *hypersensitivity* reactions than the whole molecule.

Percoll® A colloidal suspension of silica used in isopyknic *density gradient centrifugation*.

perforin Protein found in granules of cytolytic cells such as *cytotoxic T lymphocytes*, in which it is formed during *immune responses*, and in *NK cells*, in which it is present constitutively. Normally found as a monomer that has no cytolytic activity, but on contact with target cells, the granules fuse with the *lymphocyte* plasma membrane, the perforins are released and, in the presence of Ca^{2+}, they form amphipathic ring polymers of 12–18 molecules which resemble the *membrane attack complex* of *complement*. These insert into the membrane of the target cell causing lysis of the latter.

periarteriolar lymphatic sheath (PALS) The *thymus dependent area* of the white pulp of the *spleen* q.v.

peripheral lymphoid organs Those lymphoid organs that are not essential to the ontogeny of the *immune response*, i.e. *spleen, lymph nodes, tonsils, Peyer's patches*. Cf. *central lymphoid organs*.

peripheral sensitization In *transplantation immunology*, the postulated *priming* of *lymphocytes* at the actual site of the graft, as opposed to central sensitization in which *antigens* from the graft travel from it to the organs of immunity.

peritoneal exudate cells Any cells present in a peritoneal exudate. After injection into the peritoneal cavity of animals of substances such as thioglycollate, glycogen, paraffin oil, peptone or microorganisms such as *BCG*, an exudate composed mainly of *neutrophil leucocytes* forms within a few hours and this is replaced a few days later by an exudate composed mainly of *macrophages* and *lymphocytes*. However, the yield of the different cell types varies greatly between species and between stimuli and it may be noted that the cells obtained by lavage of the peritoneal cavity of mice, into which no irritant materials have been inoculated, are mainly macrophages.

pernicious anaemia *Autoimmune disease* of man characterized by atrophic gastritis with achlorhydria and lack of gastric intrinsic factor which leads to failure of absorption of dietary vitamin B_{12} and consequent megaloblastic anaemia. Sometimes associated with autoimmune *thyroiditis*. Gastric secretions and also *serum* of patients contain *autoantibodies* against intrinsic factor (70% of cases) and against an antigen present in gastric parietal cells which has been identified as the proton pump, H^+/K^+, ATPase.

peroxidase–anti-peroxidase technique (PAP technique) A variant of *enzyme labelling* techniques for detecting *antigen* or *antibody* in tissue sections by binding *immune complexes* containing horseradish peroxidase and (normally) rabbit anti peroxidase. The tissue section is incubated with rabbit antibody specific for the antigen to be detected. This is followed by an excess of anti rabbit *IgG* followed by the PAP complex. The anti rabbit IgG links the antigen-bound antibody to the PAP complexes which are then stained by incubation with a substrate, producing a coloured product. This method gives greater sensitivity than the simpler enzyme staining methods due to the multiplication effect of the PAP complex. (See Figure P1 and also *APAAP* technique.)

Peyer's patches Lymphoepithelial nodules in the submucosa of the small intestine, more prominent in the ileum (lower part) than in the jejunum. Contain *lymphocytes* including the precursors of *IgA*-producing *B cells*, *germinal centres* and *thymus dependent areas*. These *lymphoid tissues* are separated from the lumen of the intestine by a single layer of columnar epithelium (follicle associated or dome epithelium) containing specialized cells (microfold-M-cells) which take up *antigen* from the lumen and transport it into the lymphoid areas. Peyer's patches are believed to be the principal site for induction of intestinal *immune responses*.

PFC See *plaque-forming cell assay*.

pFc′ fragment A fragment produced after pepsin digestion of *IgG*. It is a noncovalently bonded dimer of the C-terminal *immunoglobulin domains* (i.e. C_H3; see C_H1 etc.) of the *Fc fragment*. Differs from the *Fc′ fragment* by retaining the basic N-terminal and C-terminal peptides of this *domain*. Cathodic electrophoretic mobility, MW 27 kD.

PHA (phytohaemagglutinins) *Lectins* extracted from the seeds (beans) of *Phaseolus vulgaris* or *P. communis*. They may be partially purified to yield a protein-rich form PHA-P or a mucoprotein-rich extract PHA-M. In soluble form they are strong *mitogens* for the *T lymphocytes* of man and mouse due to their binding affinity for N-acetyl-β-D-galactosamine residues. They also act as mitogens for *B lymphocytes* if presented to them on an insoluble matrix. Phytohaemagglutinin also causes *agglutination* of erythrocytes.

phage neutralization test An assay of *antibody* against bacteriophage. Incubation with antibody inhibits the capacity of bacteriophages to infect their host bacterium. This effect can be measured quantitatively by observing the reduction in the numbers of plaques produced by the mixture after various periods of incubation when subsequently added to a 'lawn' of bacteria. Very low levels of antibody can be detected by this technique.

phagocyte A cell that is able to ingest, and often to digest, large particles such as effete blood cells, bacteria, protozoa

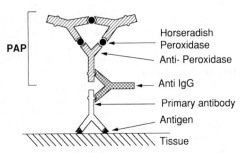

Figure P1. Peroxidase–anti-peroxidase technique.

and dead tissue cells. They are also active in ingesting foreign colloidal materials such as finely divided carbon. See *phagocytosis*. Examples of phagocytes are *macrophages, Kupffer cells,* and *neutrophil leucocytes*. See also *mononuclear phagocyte*.

phagocytosis 'cell eating'. The ingestion of cells or particles by inclusion in a cytoplasmic *phagosome* q.v. In mammals, only cells of the *mononuclear phagocyte* system and *neutrophil leucocytes* are 'professional' *phagocytes* although other cells may, on occasion, show facultative phagocytosis.

phagolysosome The product of the fusion of *lysosomes* with a *phagosome*. Materials included within it may be digested by hydrolysis. Following such digestion the vesicle may continue to function and is sometimes called a 'secondary lysosome'.

phagosome An intracellular vesicle in a *phagocyte* q.v. formed by invagination of the cell membrane and containing phagocytosed (see *phagocytosis*) material. The latter is digested by lysosomal (see *lysosome*) enzymes liberated into the vesicle following fusion of the phagosome with cytoplasmic lysosomes. The structure which results from this fusion is known as a *phagolysosome*.

pharyngeal tonsil See *tonsil*.

phycoerythrin A *fluorochrome* which emits a red fluorescence and is frequently used to label *antibodies,* especially for *double labelling* in which

one antibody is labelled with *FITC* (green) and the other with phycoerythrin (red) (e.g. a*CD3* and a*CD19*) for identifying *T cells* and *B cells*.

phytohaemagglutinins See *PHA*.

pigeon fancier's lung See *bird fancier's lung*.

pinocytosis 'cell drinking' Ingestion of fluid-containing vesicles by cells, see *endocytosis*.

PK test (Prausnitz–Küstner reaction) See *skin sensitizing antibody*.

PKA See *protein kinase A*.

PKC See *protein kinase C*.

plaque-forming cell (PFC) assay A method of importance in the development of immunology that was used to detect and enumerate *antibody* producing cells. *Primed lymphocytes* are mixed with molten Agarose® containing sheep erythrocytes (SRBC) coated with *antigen* (or SRBC themselves may be used as antigen). The Agarose® is allowed to set in a thin layer and incubated at 37°C. *Complement* is added and any cells that have secreted specific antibody are revealed by the appearance of a zone of haemolysis or plaque. The technique described reveals *IgM*-secreting cells forming direct plaques. Indirect plaques due to *IgG*-secreting cells are revealed by the addition of an anti-IgG serum. See also *Cunningham plaque technique, ELISPOT assay*.

plasma The fluid phase of blood in which the red and white blood cells are suspended.

plasma cell Cell of *B lymphocyte* lineage with a major role in antibody synthesis and secretion. The cytoplasm is basophilic, rich in RNA and protein, and packed with rough-surfaced *endoplasmic reticulum*. The nucleus is often round and eccentrically placed, with clumped chromatin giving a 'clock face' or 'cartwheel' appearance. The plasma cell is the end cell of the *B lymphocyte* line. It is the major *immunoglobulin*-secreting cell type and therefore the classical cell of *humoral immunity*. Present in *lymphoid tissue* and increased in numbers in the draining *lymph node* and at the site of entry of *antigen* following antigenic stimulation.

plasma half-life (T½) Measure of rate of catabolism of any *plasma* constituent. In immunology commonly used of the time taken for half of the *immunoglobulin* in the plasma to be catabolized.

plasma pool The quantity of *immunoglobulin* in the *plasma* per unit body weight, normally expressed as mg of immunoglobulin per kg body weight.

plasmablast *Blast cell* characterized by its prominent, clumped nuclear chromatin, and some differentiation of the *endoplasmic reticulum*, and Golgi apparatus. Precursor of the *plasma cell*.

plasmacyte See *plasma cell*.

plasmacytoma A localized tumour of *plasma cells* in contrast to *myelomatosis* which is a diffuse plasma cell tumour in *bone marrow* and elsewhere. Plasmacytomas occur rarely and spontaneously in man, outside the bone marrow in tissues such as the nasal, oral and pharyngeal mucosa and gut. The major immunological interest is that they can be induced in rats and mice (especially the BALB/c mouse strain) by intraperitoneal injection of paraffin oil, *complete Freund's adjuvant* and other substances. Many tumours producing monoclonal *immunoglobulin* of each class and subclass (see *immunoglobulin class* and

immunoglobulin subclass) have been obtained in this way and may be maintained by serial transplantation or adaptation to tissue culture. Widely used for studies on immunoglobulin biosynthesis and gene structure, as a source of *monoclonal* immunoglobulin and for fusion with *primed lymphocytes* to produce *monoclonal antibody*.

platelet (thrombocyte) A small nonnucleated 'cell' (3 μm diameter) found in mammalian blood, and derived from the megakaryocytes of *bone marrow*. It is important in blood coagulation as generator of thromboplastin on contact with foreign surfaces and is essential for haemostasis and thrombosis. Can be activated, e.g. by *TNF-α* or *eosinophil leucocyte*-derived cationic proteins to release inflammatory mediators such as *platelet activating factor, TGF-β, reactive oxygen intermediates* and arachidonic acid metabolites. Platelet activation is believed to contribute to the pathogenesis of *asthma*.

platelet activating factor (PAF; PAF acether) 1-0-hexadecyl-2-acetyl-sn-glycero-3-phosphorylcholine, a lipid released by various cells, including *platelets, mast cells* and *mononuclear phagocytes*, in the presence of *antigen*. Release may be *IgE*-mediated. Induces platelet aggregation and degranulation, and is a chemotactic factor (see *chemotaxis*), especially for *eosinophil leucocytes*. Inactivated by phospholipase A.

PMN See *polymorphonuclear leucocyte*.

pneumococcal polysaccharide Type specific antigenic polysaccharide present in the capsule of *Streptococcus pneumoniae*, its presence being related to the virulence of the organism. A *thymus independent antigen* (a *TI-2 antigen*). Each pneumococcal serotype has a structurally different polysaccharide in its capsule. These are made up of oligosaccharide repeating units, e.g. type III is composed of repeating units of glucose and glucuronic acid.

***Pneumocystis carinii* pneumonia** (PCP) Opportunistic infection in *immu-*

nosuppressed subjects caused by the ubiquitous protozoon *Pneumocystis carinii*. One of the characteristic signs of *AIDS* where infection can further reduce peripheral *CD4 lymphocyte* counts.

PNH cells Erythrocytes from patients with *paroxysmal nocturnal haemoglobinuria* (q.v.). These cells lyse spontaneously at slightly acid pH. The lytic activity of *complement* for PNH cells is abnormally high, this is due to the absence of integral control proteins (e.g. *CD59*) on the erythrocytes which prevent the insertion of the *membrane attack complex*.

poison ivy hypersensitivity *Hypersensitivity* (especially *contact hypersensitivity*) to the poison ivy plant (*Rhus toxicodendron*) which grows in North America, but not in Europe. The *allergens* of poison ivy have been isolated and are catechols. Lesions are those of *delayed-type hypersensitivity* (*type IV hypersensitivity reaction*).

pokeweed mitogen This term covers five (Pa 1–5) *mitogens* q.v. obtained from *Phytolacca americana*. Pa 1 is active for both *T lymphocytes* and *B lymphocytes*, but Pa 2, 3 and 4 only activate T lymphocytes.

poliomyelitis vaccines (a) Sabin vaccine, the oral poliomyelitis *vaccine* now in general use, contains live attenuated strains of the three types of poliomyelitis virus. These multiply in the gastrointestinal tract and stimulate good blood *antibody* production and local gut *immunity*. Given in three oral doses. It has largely superseded: (b) Salk vaccine, prepared from formalin-killed poliovirus and given by three subcutaneous injections.

pollen hypersensitivity *Immediate hypersensitivity* (*type I hypersensitivity reaction*) occurring in *atopic* subjects, usually on inhalation of pollens. Characterized by respiratory symptoms, *hay fever* or *asthma*. Many pollens may cause symptoms, especially Timothy grass pollen in Britain and ragweed in USA. Diagnosed by *skin tests* using pollen extracts.

polyacrylamide gel electrophoresis (PAGE) A high resolution electrophoresis technique carried out in a transparent synthetic acrylamide polymer gel. The gel acts as a molecular sieve and, in the presence of sodium dodecyl sulphate (hence SDS-PAGE), the mobility of a protein molecule is inversely proportional to the log of its molecular weight. If the SDS is omitted, the charge of the protein molecules as well as their molecular weight affect their mobility.

polyclonal activators General term for substances that activate many clones of *lymphocytes*, in contrast to *antigen* which activates only a restricted number of clones. See *mitogen* and *lectin*.

polymerase chain reaction (PCR) Simple, rapid and sensitive method for the *in vitro* amplification of specific DNA sequences. A thermostable DNA polymerase is used in combination with template DNA and primers in repetitive cycles of (a) denaturation of the double-stranded template DNA; (b) annealing of primers; and (c) polymerization. The primers are short oligonucleotides complementary to sequences on the template DNA that flank, and delineate, the sequence to be amplified. The method is so sensitive that a single DNA molecule can serve as the initial template and can be used, for example, to extract single copy genes from genomic DNA. The PCR technique in its various forms has found widespread use in gene cloning, DNA sequencing and site-directed mutagenesis, in the diagnosis of infectious disease and in forensic science.

polymorphonuclear leucocyte Synonym for *neutrophil leucocyte* which, in its mature form, has a multilobed nucleus though other cell types, e.g. *eosinophil leucocytes* may also have multilobed nuclei.

polyvalent antiserum *Antiserum* containing *antibodies* against many *antigens*, e.g. rabbit anti human *globulin* may contain antibodies against 20–30 *serum* globulins.

polyvalent vaccine A *vaccine* containing *protective antigens* derived from several strains of a single species of pathogenic organism. Cf. *mixed vaccines*.

positive selection The process which ensures that mature *antigen*-reactive *T lymphocytes* will only recognize (see *recognition*) foreign antigenic peptide when presented in association with a self *major histocompatibility complex* (MHC) molecule (see *MHC restriction*). This occurs during development in the *thymus* because T cells expressing T cell receptors (see *TCR*) capable of interacting with self MHC molecules are rescued from *programmed cell death*. Positive selection also occurs in *germinal centre B cells* which recognize their specific antigen in the form of *immune complexes* on *follicular dendritic cells* provided that accessory molecules (e.g. *CD40L*) are also present. High *affinity* B cells are thus rescued from programmed cell death.

post-capillary venules Small vessels through which blood flows after leaving the capillaries and before reaching the veins. It is between the endothelial cells of post-capillary venules (rather than capillaries) that most *leucocytes* migrate into inflammatory sites. The *high endothelial venules* (q.v.) of *lymph nodes* are specialized post-capillary venules through which the *recirculating pool* of *lymphocytes* pass from blood to *lymph*, see *lymphocyte recirculation*.

PPD (purified protein derivative) A mixture of proteins, purified from *Mycobacterium tuberculosis*, and employed in the *tuberculin test* (*Mantoux test*) as a diagnostic reagent for detecting sensitization by, or infection with, M. tuberculosis. PPD is a powerful activator of *T lymphocytes* from tuberculin-sensitive individuals *in vitro* and also a *mitogen* for *B lymphocytes* in mice acting mainly on differentiated cells to induce *immunoglobulin* production.

Prausnitz–Küstner reaction (PK test) See *skin sensitizing antibody*.

pre-B lymphocyte (pre-B cell) *B cell* precursor which has developed from a *pro-B lymphocyte*, and which has begun to rearrange the *heavy chain* genes of *immunoglobulin* and to synthesize μ chains. The latter associate with *surrogate light chains* and may be expressed with them on the cell surface. When synthesis of functional *light chains* begins and the cell assembles *IgM* molecules, it becomes a B lymphocyte.

pre-T lymphocyte (pre-T cell) *Bone marrow*-derived precursor of *T lymphocyte* which has not yet undergone *education* or development in the *thymus*.

precipitation In immunology, the formation of a visible *immune complex* on the addition of soluble *antibody* to soluble *antigen*. Such complexes are detected in the test tube as a sediment and in agar gels (see *gel diffusion test*) as a white line appearing where the antigen and antibody interact. Precipitation does not take place in all proportions of antibody–antigen mixtures even though combination *has* taken place. Also, special conditions may be necessary to effect precipitation with *immunoglobulins* of the various classes of vertebrates, e.g. a high salt concentration is required for avian sera. See *antigen excess, antibody excess, optimal proportions*.

precipitin *Antibody* which reacts with *antigen* to form a precipitate. See *precipitation*.

precipitin test A test in which the reaction of *antibody* with a soluble *antigen* is detected by the formation of a visible precipitate. See *quantitative precipitin test, gel diffusion test, precipitation*.

premunition (premunity; non-sterile immunity) A state of *protective immunity* maintained by the persistence of small numbers of the pathogenic organism within the body. Loss of these organisms, e.g. due to drug treatment, may result in a return to susceptibility and acute re-infection. Recrudescence of the premunizing infection in virulent form may also follow debility or *splenectomy*. Premunity is especially seen in diseases caused by blood-borne protozoa, e.g. babesiosis of cattle and dogs, but may also be the basis of the *tuberculin test* response in man.

primary allergen In cases of *cross sensitivity* q.v. describes the substance which *primed* the patient.

primary antibody In double layer staining techniques (such as *double layer immunofluorescence*) for detection of tissue or cell-surface *antigens*, and in the *ELISA* assay, the primary antibody, which is specific for the antigen in question and unconjugated (see *conjugate*), is applied first and the excess washed away. A conjugated (i.e. labelled) *secondary antibody* is then added. This is an anti *immunoglobulin* which binds to the primary antibody thus allowing detection and localization of the antigen.

primary follicle See *lymphoid follicle*.

primary granule See *azurophil granule*.

primary immune response The response of the animal body to an *antigen* on the first occasion that it encounters it. Characteristically, low levels of *antibody* are produced slowly but *priming* of the *lymphoid tissues* allows a *secondary immune response* (cf.) to be evoked on subsequent *challenge*. Responses of *cell-mediated immunity* follow a similar pattern.

primary interaction A term used to describe the initial binding of an *antibody* to an *antigen* whether or not this gives rise to a secondary effect such as *precipitation* or *complement activation*. Tests that measure primary antigen–antibody interactions are the *Farr test, equilibrium dialysis*, fluorescence quenching, fluorescence polarization and tests employing other techniques such as differential centrifugation or electrophoresis to separate bound from unbound antibody molecules.

primary lymphoid tissues Synonym for *central lymphoid organs*.

primary lysosome A *lysosome* prior to fusion with a *phagosome*.

primary nodule See *lymphoid follicle*.

primed (1) Of a whole animal: Exposed to *antigen* in such a way that the antigen makes contact with the *lymphoid tissue* so that the appropriate responsive cells are activated. Further contact of a primed host with antigen usually results in a vigorous, rapid, *secondary immune response*. (2) Of *lymphocytes*: A primed lymphocyte is one that has been specifically activated in respect of a given antigen and can divide and give rise to *effector lymphocytes* and *memory cells*. The effector lymphocytes are either *B cells* which synthesize *immunoglobulin*, or *T cells* which mediate the reactions of *cell-mediated immunity*.

primed lymphocyte *Lymphocyte*, *primed* (q.v.) specifically to an *antigen*.

priming (1) Of *immune responses*: The events that follow initial contact with *antigen*. See *primed*. (2) Of *neutrophil leucocytes*: Addition of a stimulus (e.g. *lipopolysaccharide, TNF-α, GM-CSF*, chemotactic factors) at a dose too low to stimulate an *oxidative metabolic burst*, but which primes the cell so that on addition of a second stimulus, which may not be identical to the first, a much larger metabolic burst is obtained than in unprimed cells.

priming dose The first dose of any *antigen* given to an animal in order to stimulate an *immune response*.

private determinant (private epitope) An *epitope* which is found only on the product of a single allele of an *allogeneic* system. Commonly used of *alloantigens* of the *HLA histocompatibility system*.

privileged sites Sites in the body lacking normal lymphatic drainage and into which *antigens*, or tissue grafts, can be placed without stimulating an *immune response*, e.g. the central nervous system, the anterior chamber of the eye, and the cheek-pouch of the hamster.

pro-B lymphocyte The most immature identifiable precursor of the *B lympho-*

cyte. Expresses *surrogate light chains*, receptors for *IL-7* and membrane *CD19*.

processing See *antigen processing*.

programmed cell death Death of cells due to activation of a genetic programme that instructs the cell to commit suicide. Requires new gene expression. Frequently takes the form of *apoptosis*, but the latter does not always involve gene expression by the dying cell. Important generally in developmental biology and, in immunology, in selection of *lymphocytes* during maturation. Some of the genes involved are known, e.g. *fas* (see *Fas*). Other genes, e.g. *bcl-2*, are necessary for rescue of developing haemopoietic cells from cell death.

properdin (P; Factor P) Protein of the *alternative pathway* of *complement activation*. Exists in the circulation as a mixture of polymers (monomer 53 kD). Binds and stabilizes alternative pathway *C3 convertase* and *C5 convertase* preventing their spontaneous dissociation.

prophylactic immunization The use of *immunization* to prevent disease. Usually, but not always, *active immunization* which has a longer lasting effect than *passive immunization*.

propidium iodide A fluorescent dye that binds to DNA. Used in cell cycle studies and also as a measure of *apoptosis*, since an altered *flow cytometry* profile is associated with DNA fragmentation, a characteristic of apoptotic cells.

prostaglandins Biologically active lipids generated by the action of cycloxygenases on arachidonic acid (cf. *leukotrienes*, which are generated by lipoxygenase action). There is a large number of prostaglandins, which have a variety of activities as inflammatory mediators. The actions of different prostaglandins may be mutually antagonistic. *Mast cells* release PGI$_2$ (prostacyclin), a potent inhibitor of *platelet* aggregation, a vasodilator, and inhibitor of release of leukotrienes. They also release PGD$_2$, a smooth muscle constrictor. Other cycloxygenase products released during anaphylactic reactions (see *anaphylaxis*) include thromboxane A$_2$, which causes platelet aggregation, PGF$_2$, a smooth muscle constrictor, and PGE$_2$, a smooth muscle relaxant and vasodilator.

proteasome A proteolytic complex that degrades proteins within the cytosol (that is, the cytoplasm other than organelles and membranes) and nuclear proteins. Implicated in *antigen processing*. See Figure A2.

protective antigens Those *antigens* of a pathogenic microorganism that, if given alone, will stimulate an *immune response* capable of providing protection against infection by that organism.

protective immunity *Non-specific immunity* and/or *specific immunity* that is protective, e.g. against a pathogenic microorganism, in contrast to *immunity* stimulated by an experimental *antigen* such as *ovalbumin*, or by an internal antigen of the pathogen. See *protective antigen*.

protein A (staphylococcal protein A; SPA; SpA) Monomeric protein from the cell wall of *Staphylococcus aureus*. Binds to the C$_H$2 and C$_H$3 (see *C$_H$1* etc.) domains from man (IgG1, 2 and 4; see *IgG1* etc.), guinea pig (IgG1 and 2), mouse (IgG2a and 2b) and rabbit. Does not bind human IgG3. Each protein A molecule can bind to two *IgG* molecules. Protein A may inhibit *Fc receptor*-mediated (but not *C3b* receptor-mediated) *phagocytosis* by binding to the *Fc fragment* of opsonizing *antibody* (see *opsonin*). The ability of protein A to bind IgG makes it a valuable reagent for affinity purification of IgG and for the detection of IgG *immune complexes*. Protein A is also a *polyclonal activator* for *B cells*.

protein G A protein found in the cell wall of Group C streptococci. It binds to the *Fc fragment* of all subclasses of human *IgG* (unlike *protein A*, which does not bind human IgG3) and that of many other species, including bovine, sheep and goat IgG, which it binds more strongly than protein A. Often used as a substitute for protein A in affinity purification and immunoassays where these immunoglobulins are present.

protein kinase An enzyme that phosphorylates proteins either on serine and threonine, e.g. *protein kinase A, protein kinase C,* or on tyrosine (*protein tyrosine kinases*). Important in intracellular signalling.

protein kinase A A serine–threonine *protein kinase* activated by cyclic AMP, an important signalling molecule in most cells including those of the immune system.

protein kinase C A kinase that exists in a number of isoforms and that phosphorylates serine and threonine residues in target proteins. It is itself activated by diacylglycerol derived from cleavage of membrane lipids. Activity is frequently calcium-dependent. An important regulator of cell functions including many functions in cells of the immune system. See *G proteins.*

protein tyrosine kinase An enzyme that phosphorylates the hydroxyl group of tyrosine residues of proteins. There are numerous tyrosine kinases, many of which are involved in intracellular signalling following *ligand–receptor* binding in cells including those of the immune system.

prozone In *agglutination* and *precipitation* tests, agglutination/precipitation may not occur in the tubes containing the highest concentration of *antibody* but becomes obvious when the antibody is diluted. This absence or weakness of agglutination/precipitation in the presence of the high levels of antibody is known as a prozone. It may be due to: (a) *blocking antibody*[1] q.v.; (b) binding of antibody only to single cells or molecules, e.g. an *antibody excess* situation; or (c) non-specific inhibition by other *serum* proteins or lipids. In precipitating systems, *soluble complexes* formed in antibody excess are present in the prozone, i.e. (b).

pseudoallergic reaction Clinical state that mimics the symptoms and signs of *immediate hypersensitivity* but without evidence for an immunological mechanism. The majority of drug reactions are of this type.

PTK See *protein tyrosine kinase.*

public determinant (public epitope) An *epitope* shared by more than one gene product within an *allogeneic* system. Commonly used of *alloantigens* of the *HLA histocompatibility system.* *Antibodies* to public determinants have been used to classify HLA antigens serologically into several major *cross reactive groups* (CREGS). See also *private determinant.*

purified protein derivative See *PPD.*

purine nucleoside phosphorylase deficiency (PNP deficiency) An autosomal recessive defect due to inheritance of a mutant form of PNP. Toxic metabolites accumulate in *T cells* and there is primarily a deficiency of *cell-mediated immunity* with normal numbers of *B cells,* though *antibody* production may be impaired as a secondary effect.

Q

Qa antigens Murine *histocompatibility antigens* related in structure to *class I MHC antigen* molecules and coded for by genes distal to *H-2 D/L* and closely linked to *Tla* (see *H-2 histocompatibility system*). Identified using *alloantisera, monoclonal antibodies* and allospecific *T cells* this region has at least five loci (Qa1–5) each of which appears to have two alleles, one a null allele. May present foreign peptides to class I *MHC restricted* T cells. See Figure H1.

quantitative gel diffusion tests *Gel diffusion tests* that enable an estimate of the quantity of an *antibody*, or more usually, of an *antigen* to be made. See *single radial diffusion test*.

quantitative precipitation test *Precipitin test* in which a row of tubes is set up so that the ratio of *antibody* to *antigen* is varied (sequentially) from tube to tube. Antigen and antibody are present at *optimal proportions* in that tube in which *precipitation* occurs most rapidly and in which the precipitate is most abundant. As all of the antibody capable of forming a precipitate is precipitated in that tube, quantitative estimations of antibody in terms of protein concentration can be achieved.

R

r Abbreviation for recombinant.

R Abbreviation for *receptor*.

radial immunodiffusion test See *single radial diffusion test*.

radiation chimera See *irradiation chimera*.

radioallergosorbent test See *RAST*.

radioimmunoassay Any method of measuring *antibody* or *antigen* concentration by employing radioactively labelled reactants.

Raji cell assay *In vitro* assay to identify *immune complexes* using the Raji *B lymphocyte* tumour line. These cells have receptors for *C3b* and for the *Fc fragment* of *IgG* but no surface *immunoglobulins*. Complexes bound to their surfaces can therefore be detected using labelled anti immunoglobulin after blocking the *Fc receptors*.

RANTES (Regulation upon Activation Normal T cell Expressed and Secreted) A β *chemokine*, see Table C2.

RAST Method for measuring *IgE* antibody specific for various *allergens*. In clinical work, serum IgE *antibody* is usually measured. The *serum* is reacted with allergen-coated cellulose discs which are washed to remove non-reacting proteins. Radiolabelled anti human IgE *antiserum* is then added and this binds to the IgE antibody. Provided that the amounts of allergen and anti IgE are in excess, the radioactivity of the disc after washing is proportional to the amount of allergen-specific antibody in the serum sample. Values are expressed as arbitrary RAST units, one unit approximates to 2 ng of IgE antibody.

RCA gene family (regulators of complement activation) This group of *comp-lement* components; *Factor H, C4 binding protein* (C4bp), *CR1, decay accelerating factor, membrane cofactor protein* (MCP) and *CR2* show genetic linkage and belong to the *SCR superfamily*. The genes are located (in humans) on chromosome 1 in the G32 region, and the proteins which are involved in complement regulation (except for CR2) have arisen by a combination of gene duplication and *exon* shuffling.

reaction of identity Reaction on *gel diffusion test* plate (especially *Ouchterlony test*) which demonstrates the antigenic identity of two test solutions. The two solutions of *antigen* are placed in separate wells and allowed to diffuse towards *antibody* in a third well. If the resultant line of *precipitation* is continuous, this is known as a reaction of identity. See Figure R1.

reaction of non-identity Reaction on *gel diffusion test* plate (especially *Ouchterlony test*) which demonstrates the antigenic non-identity of two test materials. Solutions of these are each placed in a well and allowed to diffuse towards *antibody* in a third well. If two lines of *precipitation* are seen, each corresponding to one of the antigen solutions, and these lines cross, this is a reaction of non-identity. See Figure R2.

reaction of partial identity Reaction on *gel diffusion test* plate (especially

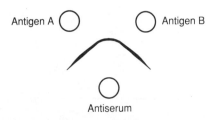

Figure R1. Reaction of identity.

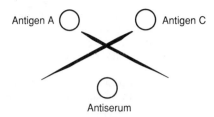

Figure R2. Reaction of non-identity.

Ouchterlony test) which demonstrates that a given test substance shares *epitopes* with a second substance but has other epitopes which are not shared. The *antigens* are each placed in wells and allowed to diffuse towards *antibody* in a third well. The resultant line of *precipitation* is continuous, because of the shared epitope, but has a spur formed by the unshared epitope. See Figure R3.

reactive haemolysis Lysis of unsensitized (i.e. with no attached antibody) erythrocytes initiated by a stable complex of the activated *C5* and *C6* components of *complement*. Phenomenon shown especially by *acute phase sera*.

reactive nitrogen intermediates Free radical gases which are made up of nitrogen and oxygen, including NO, NO_2^-, NO_3^- and $HNOO^-$. They are derived from the guanidino nitrogen of L-arginine and are mediators of a variety of biological functions. See *nitric oxide*.

reactive oxygen intermediates (ROI) Reactive metabolites of molecular oxygen generated in *phagocytes* via the NADPH oxidase/cytochrome b electron donor system (see *chronic granulomatous disease*). The major species are superoxide (O_2^-), hydrogen peroxide (H_2O_2) and hydroxyl radical (OH).

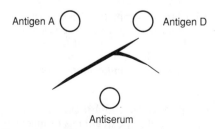

Figure R3. Reaction of partial identity.

These are generated following *phagocytosis* and are rapidly microbicidal.

reagin (reaginic antibody) Term historically used to describe *antibody* of the *IgE* class which fixes to tissue cells of the same species so that, on reaction with *antigen, histamine* and other vasoactive agents are released.

receptor (R) Macromolecule, usually a protein, which contains a site capable of selectively combining, with a varying degree of specificity, with complementary molecules known as *ligands*. In immunology, usually refers to cell surface molecules, e.g. *membrane immunoglobulin* receptors for *antigen* on *B lymphocytes*, the T cell receptor (*TCR*), *cytokine* receptors, etc., though some receptors, e.g. for corticosteroids, are intracellular. The term 'receptor' usually refers to molecules with specific binding sites at which binding is followed by transduction of a signal across the membrane and a response on the part of the cell.

recirculating pool All the *lymphocytes* that continuously recirculate between blood and *lymph*, see *lymphocyte recirculation*.

recirculation See *lymphocyte recirculation*.

recognition Term used for the interactions by which cells (or molecules such as *antibody*) discriminate between materials in their environment. Recognition may be a property of specific *receptors* by which molecules are selectively bound (e.g. *antigen* by antibody), or may be relatively non-specific. Recognition at cell surface receptors is usually followed by activation of cellular function, for example the activation of antibody synthesis in *B lymphocytes* following cell surface binding of antigens.

recombinant strains Strains of animals (e.g. mice, sheep) in which the genes in the parental strains have either been reassorted (i.e. recombined) by breeding techniques (to give recombinant inbred strains) or altered by direct DNA manipulation. Recombinant inbred (RI) strains provide large numbers of virtually genetically uniform and homozygous mice in which the effects of reassorting various parental genes (e.g. *heavy chain* genes) can be studied.

recombinant vaccine *Subunit vaccines* based on proteins derived from recombinant DNA techniques. The gene for a target *antigen* that is to be incorporated in a *vaccine*, is first identified, then cloned. The cDNA is then introduced into a suitable expression plasmid which is then transfected into a cell line (bacterial, yeast, insect or mammalian). The transfected cells produce large amounts of the antigen which can then be purified for use as vaccine. This process produces highly purified vaccines at relatively low cost.

red pulp of spleen See *spleen*.

regulators of complement activation gene family See *RCA gene family*.

rejection See *immunological rejection*.

repeating units Term used of macromolecular structures, especially *antigens*, in which an identical configuration occurs repeatedly, e.g. the polysaccharide cell wall antigens of Gram negative bacteria are repeated along the length of the organism. *Pneumococcal polysaccharide* type III consists of a repeating structure of -β-1,4-glucose-β-1,3-glucuronic acid. Antigens with a repeating unit structure are frequently *thymus independent antigens*, see *TI-2 antigen*.

repertoire (1) The number of different *antibody* or *TCR* (T cell receptor), *variable region* sequences produced by the immune system of a given species. (2) The number of different *epitopes* recognized by all the antibodies or T cell receptors produced by the immune system of a species.
These two definitions are not synonymous since there is redundancy within the system, i.e. several antibody molecules or T cell receptors with different variable regions are able to recognize the same epitope. The number of different epitope-recognizing *receptors* on *B cells* or *T cells* produced by an individual animal or human at any one time is much less than the number that the immune system is capable of producing – the 'potential repertoire'.

resident macrophage *Macrophage* present at a site in the absence of a known eliciting stimulus.

respiratory burst The increase in anaerobic glycolytic metabolism and oxygen consumption which occurs following activation of *phagocytes*, e.g. *neutrophil leucocytes*, by chemotactic factors (see *chemotaxis*), *phagocytosis*, etc. and which is accompanied by enhanced NADPH oxidase activity leading to generation of microbicidal *reactive oxygen intermediates*.

restriction fragment length polymorphism analysis (RFLP analysis) The use of restriction endonucleases to cleave DNA at defined sites (restriction sites) thus producing an array of DNA fragments containing various genes. Allelic genes may vary in their expression of particular restriction sites, leading to variations in the length of the DNA fragments produced. Fragments containing known genes can be identified by *Southern blotting*. In *histocompatibility testing*, restriction fragment length polymorphism can be correlated with defined serological (e.g. HLA-DR/DQ) and cellular (e.g. HLA-DW) specificities (see *HLA class II locus*). For this purpose, a single restriction enzyme (TAQ1) and cDNA probes specific for HLA-DRβ, -DQβ and -DQα are used.

reticular cells Cells that, together with reticular fibres, make up the framework or stroma of *lymphoid tissues* such as the *spleen* and *lymph nodes* and of the *bone marrow*.

reticular dysgenesis The most complete form of severe combined immunodeficiency syndrome (*SCID*) in which there is a defect of maturation of all *leucocytes*, i.e. *lymphocytes*, *granulocytes* and *monocytes*.

reticuloendothelial blockade Administration of large quantities of inert particles, e.g. colloidal carbon or iron, by the intravenous or peritoneal routes with the aim of saturating most of the actively phagocytosing (see *phagocytosis*) cells of the *mononuclear phagocyte* system so that they are temporarily incapable of further phagocytosis.

reticuloendothelial system A term coined by Aschoff (1913) to describe a system of cells that had the ability to take up and retain certain dyes and particles when these were injected into the living animal. It has been replaced by the term *mononuclear phagocyte* system q.v.

reticulosis See *lymphoma*.

reverse immunoblotting A technique for the analysis of the clonality of an *antibody* response. *Serum* or other fluid containing antibody is separated by *isoelectric focusing* (IEF) and the molecules are then transferred electrophoretically to a membrane of nitrocellulose or other material to which the antibodies bind in a pattern identical to that originally in the IEF gel (the 'blot'). The pattern of specific antibody on the membrane is revealed by incubating with radiolabelled *antigen*. Since each clone of *B cells* produces a unique pattern of antibody on an IEF gel (the *clonotype*), the number of clones responding and changes in the behaviour of individual clones can be observed. See also *immunoblotting*.

reverse passive Arthus reaction Reaction produced by injecting precipitating (see *precipitation*) *antibody* into the skin of an animal followed by intravenous injection of the corresponding *antigen* after a delay (usually of 30 minutes–2 hours). Thus the normal situation of antibody diffusing from the blood to the tissues and the antigen from the tissues to the blood has been reversed. Often used in the study of the effect of *Arthus reactions* on joints (i.e. antibody is injected into the joints). See also *passive Arthus reaction*.

RFLP analysis See *restriction fragment length polymorphism analysis*.

Rh group (Rhesus group) See *Rhesus blood group system*.

Rhesus blood group system Human *blood group* system so named because *antibody* produced in rabbits injected with rhesus monkey erythrocytes reacted with human Rhesus blood group *antigens*. The Rhesus blood group system is genetically complex. The most important erythrocyte antigen is that known as the D-antigen. Antibodies against Rhesus antigens do not occur naturally in serum, but *anti-D* antibodies may be produced after transfusion of a Rhesus (D)-negative person with Rhesus (D)-positive blood, and in a Rhesus (D)-negative mother who bears a Rhesus (D)-positive child. This may give rise to a risk of *transfusion reactions* on further transfusion, or of *erythroblastosis fetalis* in a subsequent baby.

rheumatoid arthritis Chronic inflammatory polyarthritis with systemic disturbances; toxic febrile illness, anaemia, enlargement of *lymph nodes*. More common in women than in men. Synovia of joints are swollen and infiltrated with *granulomata* containing *plasma cells*, *lymphocytes*, *macrophages* and *germinal centres*. Lesions in other connective tissues throughout the body are also seen. A putative *autoimmune disease* although evidence for autoimmune pathogenesis is not good. Serum contains *rheumatoid factor* and, in a minority of cases, *anti nuclear antibody* q.v. In 80% of cases there is an association with HLA-DR1 and HLA-DR4 (see *HLA class II locus*). See also *collagen induced arthritis* and *adjuvant arthritis*.

rheumatoid factor *Autoantibody*, primarily of *IgM* isotype, directed against aggregated *IgG*. Found in patients who have aggressive forms of *rheumatoid arthritis*. Detected by *Rose–Waaler* test or latex agglutination test (a *passive agglutination test*). The factor is thus diagnostically useful.

rhodamines A group of red fluorescent dyes, some of which are used for labelling proteins for use in *immunofluorescence* techniques, e.g. lissamine rhodamine, *tetramethylrhodamine isothiocyanate*, rhodamine B isothiocyanate.

rhodopsin superfamily A family of *Type III transmembrane proteins* which span the membrane seven times. The N-terminus is extracellular and the C-terminus cytoplasmic (see Figure T3). These proteins transduce signals by activating trimeric *G proteins* (GTP-binding proteins) and signal transduction can be blocked with pertussis toxin. Many chemotaxis receptors (for *C5a*, *formyl peptides*, *IL-8* and other *chemokines*) belong to this family. Many other members are found in the central nervous system.

RNI See *reactive nitrogen intermediates.*

ROI See *reactive oxygen intermediates.*

Rose–Waaler test *Passive agglutination test* in which sera are titrated against sheep erythrocytes coated with *gamma globulin*. The sera of a high proportion of cases of *rheumatoid arthritis* contain *antibodies* against *IgG* whose conformation has been altered, e.g. by heating or by combination with *antigen*, so that *hidden determinants* are exposed. This antibody, known as *rheumatoid factor*, *agglutinates* the gamma globulin-coated sheep erythrocytes.

rosette Cluster of erythrocytes round a *leucocyte* or other cell. See *EAC-rosette forming cell, E-rosette forming cell.*

runt disease Disease which develops after injection of *allogeneic lymphocytes* into immunologically immature experimental animals. Characterized by loss of weight, failure to thrive, diarrhoea, splenomegaly and often death. An example of a *graft-versus-host reaction.*

S

S-locus Murine 'serum substance' locus (*Ss*), so-called because it controls quantitative variations in S-protein, the murine equivalent of *C4*.

S-protein See *S-locus*.

salt precipitation Precipitation of *serum* proteins in solutions of salts such as sodium sulphate or ammonium sulphate. *Globulins* are precipitated at lower concentrations of such salts than is *albumin*. Euglobulins are precipitated at very low ionic strength. Used as a crude method for separation of serum proteins.

sandwich immunofluorescence An *indirect immunofluorescence* (or *enzyme labelling*) technique for the detection of *antibody* or antibody-producing cells in tissue sections or smears. A first layer of *antigen* is applied and allowed to react with the antibody in the section. This is followed by a second layer of *fluorochrome-* or enzyme-labelled antibody specific for the antigen. Thus the antigen is 'sandwiched' between two layers of antibody and can be detected by fluorescence or production of a coloured product. See Figure I6. A similar method is used in some *ELISA* assays to measure the concentration of antigen in solution. For best results, two *monoclonal antibodies* are used, specific for different *epitopes* on the same antigen.

sandwich technique Labelling tests in which a reagent is sandwiched between two layers of the same material the first of which is the substance being tested for. Examples are *sandwich immunofluorescence* (q.v.) and some types of *ELISA* assay.

scavenger receptor A *Type II transmembrane protein* (trimeric) found on *macrophages*. There are two forms of different molecular weights. They bind a number of modified proteins such as acetyl-LDL and maleyl-*HSA* and may have a general role in scavenging modified proteins.

scavenger receptor superfamily A number of proteins other than the *scavenger receptor* have extracellular domains of the scavenger receptor type. They include *CD5* and *CD6*.

SCID (severe combined immunodeficiency) A rare *immunodeficiency* state in infants presenting early with severe infections, diarrhoea and failure to thrive. Both *humoral immunity* and *cell-mediated immunity* are defective. There are various forms, e.g. (a) X-linked SCID in which there is a complete absence of *T cells* and T cell precursors but functional *B cells* are present, this form may be associated with mutations in the gene for the γ chain of *IL-2R*; (b) autosomal recessive forms including *adenosine deaminase deficiency*; and (c) in some cases, particular chains of the *CD3* molecule are absent. The disease can be corrected by *bone marrow* transplantation, suggesting a *stem cell* defect (involving T cell precursors prior to migration to the *thymus*). See also *bare lymphocyte syndrome* and *ZAP-70*.

SCID mouse (severe combined immunodeficiency mouse) A mouse homozygous for a recessive mutation (*scid*) on chromosome 16. Such mice have low numbers of both *B cells* and *T cells*, lack *immunoglobulin* in their *serum* and are deficient in both *humoral immunity* and *cell-mediated immunity*. Both T and B lymphocytes have a defective capacity to rearrange the genes coding for antigen *receptors*.

SCR See *short consensus repeat*.

SCR superfamily (short consensus repeat superfamily) A superfamily some of whose members are membrane proteins, others soluble proteins and many have functions within the *complement* system. The superfamily is characterized by the presence of *short consensus repeats* (SCR) which are disulphide-bonded repeating loops of about 60 residues. It includes complement receptors *CR1* and *CR2*, *Factor B*, *Factor H*, *C2*, etc. Some proteins not associated with complement (e.g. *selectins*) also may contain SRC loops.

SDS-PAGE See *polyacrylamide gel electrophoresis*.

second set rejection The *immunological rejection* of a graft by a host that has already rejected (see *first set rejection*), either tissue from the same donor, or tissue carrying similar *histocompatibility antigens*. Second set rejection is much more rapid than is first set rejection and in this resembles a *secondary immune response*.

secondary allergen The substance that produces the symptoms in cases of *cross sensitivity* and which may, superficially, appear to be unrelated to the *primary allergen* q.v.

secondary antibody A labelled anti immunoglobulin used for detecting the presence of a *primary antibody*. In double layer staining techniques (such as *double layer immunofluorescence*) for the detection of tissue or cell-surface *antigens*, an unlabelled (i.e. unconjugated, see *conjugate*) antigen-specific primary antibody is first applied. After any excess of this has been washed away, the secondary antibody is added. This binds to the primary antibody thus allowing detection and localization of the antigen by visualization of the label.

secondary follicle *Lymphoid follicle* that contains a *germinal centre*. More frequently observed in *secondary immune response* than in *primary immune response*, hence name.

secondary granule See *specific granule*.

secondary immune response Response of the immune system to an *antigen* to which it has already been *primed* (see *primary immune response*) and therefore has memory. There is very rapid production of large amounts of *antibody* over a few days followed by a slow exponential fall. The response of *cell-mediated immunity* follows a similar pattern. See also *second set rejection* and *negative phase*.

secondary lymphoid tissues Synonym for *peripheral lymphoid organs*.

secondary lysosome See *phagolysosome*.

secretory IgA The form of *IgA* found in external body secretions such as intestinal mucus, *colostrum*, milk, saliva, sweat and tears; mainly in the form of a dimer with *secretory piece* bound to it. Thus distinct from that found in the *serum*, which has no secretory piece and, in humans, is predominantly monomeric.

secretory piece Polypeptide of molecular weight 60 kD found attached to dimers of the secretory form of *IgA* (see *secretory IgA*). Structurally unrelated to *immunoglobulins* and synthesized by epithelial cells in the gut, lung, mammary or other secretory tissues, not the *plasma cells* that synthesize the immunoglobulin. Has strong *affinity* for mucus thus prolonging retention of IgA on mucous surfaces. May also inhibit the destruction of IgA by enzymes in the digestive tract. It is part of a larger molecule, a *receptor* for polymeric immunoglobulin on the surface of certain epithelial cells. The receptor binds to IgA and transports it through the cell after *endocytosis*. The receptor is then cleaved, releasing IgA with the remaining part of the molecule (the secretory piece) still attached, into the lumen of the gut, mammary gland or other organ.

selectins A family of cell adhesion molecules. *Type I transmembrane proteins* containing an N-terminal C-type *lectin* domain, and thus capable of binding to carbohydrates, together with an epidermal growth factor-like domain and a variable number of *SCR superfamily* domains. They mediate the initial adhesion of *leucocytes* to vascular endothelium by low-*affinity* interactions, and slow the cells up, causing them to roll along the side of the vessel. The leucocytes then become bound in a second step mediated by *integrin superfamily* proteins, and migrate through the vessel wall. Soluble selectins shed from cells may bind to their ligands and thus inhibit adhesion of the cell-type from which they were derived. There are three known selectins:

(a) **L-selectin** (CD62L). Expressed on most leucocytes. Binds to sialylated glycoproteins. Itself carries sialyl Lewis x (*CD15*) which is recognized by E-selectin, and this L-selectin–E-selectin interaction allows binding of *neutrophil leucocytes* to endothelium, but not of *lymphocytes*. L-selectin also mediates binding of lymphocytes to *high endothelial venules* and other endothelia possibly by binding to *GlyCAM-1*. L-selectin (like other selectins) is rapidly shed from the cell surface after activation, which may assist leucocyte detachment.

(b) **E-selectin** (CD62E; ELAM-1). Expressed on vascular endothelia 4–6 hours after activation with *lipopolysaccharide*, *IL-1* or *TNF-α* but not on unactivated endothelia. Mediates attachment of neutrophil leucocytes and *monocytes*. Binds sialyl Lewis x.

(c) **P-selectin** (CD62P). Stored in secretory granules but not on the surface of unactivated vascular endothelium. On stimulation with thrombin or *histamine*, is released to the surface within seconds. Allows transient attachment of neutrophils and monocytes, and is then internalized, its adhesive role being taken over by E-selectin. Binds to sialyl Lewis x.

See also Table A2.

selective theories of the immune response Theories which propose that *lymphocytes*, before any exposure to an *antigen*, are already pre-programmed with the information necessary to make a specific response of *humoral immunity* or *cell-mediated immunity* to it. On contact with an antigen, *B lymphocytes* or *T lymphocytes* with receptors specific for that antigen are stimulated to produce *antibody* or a cell-mediated immune response. The best known examples are Ehrlich's side chain hypothesis, Jerne's selection hypothesis and Burnet's *clonal selection theory* (q.v.). The form of selective theory proposed by Sir MacFarlane Burnet is now known to be essentially correct. The mechanism for generation of the large *repertoire* of antibodies and T cell receptors (*TCR*) required by it is now understood in considerable detail from studies on the molecular structure of germline *immunoglobulin genes* and *TCR genes* and the *translocation* events that generate large numbers of *variable region* sequences by the random recombination of *V exons, D exons,* and *J exons.* Cf. *instructive hypotheses of antibody production.*

self antigen See *autoantigen.*

self-cure In animals infested with intestinal nematodes the suddenly initiated, and thereafter exponential, expulsion from the intestine of the majority of the population of worms. It starts some 10 days after initial establishment of the infestation and may result from an *immune response* by the host. This is probably of the *immediate hypersensitivity* type causing release of vasoactive substances (see *vascular permeability factors*) from *mast cells* in the gut wall.

self tolerance *Immunological tolerance* to *autoantigens.* Such tolerance to self antigens accessible to the *lymphoid tissues,* is thought to be acquired normally during fetal life (see *negative selection*).

sensitization Administration of *antigen* to provoke an *immune response,* so that, on later *challenge¹*, a more vigorous *secondary immune response* will ensue. Used especially in context of an initial dose of antigen given in order to provoke a *hypersensitivity* reaction on subsequent challenge.

septic shock A severe, generalized, potentially lethal reaction following exposure to *lipopolysaccharide* (LPS) or other bacterial products. Characterized by shock, hypotension, fever and leucopenia. The lesions may be largely due to the presence of high and toxic levels of *TNF-α* and *IL-1* released from cells as a response to LPS or related substances. See also *endotoxin shock*.

sequestered antigen Any *antigen* or *epitope* which is hidden from contact with immunologically competent cells and thus cannot stimulate an *immune response*. Antigens in certain *privileged sites* may be sequestered from the immune system. Release of antigen, e.g. as a result of injury, may result in a response of *autoimmunity*.

serial dilutions The progressive dilution of a reagent in a row of tubes so that the first tube contains the largest amount of reagent and the last tube the smallest. See also *doubling dilution*.

serology The study of, or diagnostic application of, the reactions of *antigens* with *antibodies* *in vitro*.

serotherapy Injection of *antisera* or *antibodies* (e.g. *gamma globulin*) derived from them to produce *passive immunity* for the prophylaxis or treatment of infectious diseases. See *passive immunization*.

serotonin (5-hydroxytryptamine, 5HT) Causes smooth muscle contraction, increased vascular permeability and vasoconstriction of larger vessels. Found in *platelets* and *mast cells*. Released in *anaphylactic* reactions in rabbit but there is no direct evidence that it has a role in human anaphylaxis. It is also an important neurotransmitter.

serprocidin Serprocidins are a family of 25–29 kD proteins which share sequence homology with serine proteases and some of which have strong proteolytic activity. Found chiefly in *neutrophil leucocytes*, but also in some *macrophages*. Have antimicrobial activity.

serum Fluid expressed from a blood clot as it contracts after coagulation of the blood. The essential difference between *plasma* and serum is that the latter does not contain fibrinogen. Serum is more commonly used than is plasma in immunological procedures because there is no danger of a clot forming when other materials are added to it.

serum hepatitis (hepatitis B) Serum hepatitis, which often has a long incubation period of 2–5 months, occasionally follows transfer of *serum* or other biological fluids from one human being to another. Hazard of blood transfusion and of *passive transfer* tests.

serum sickness A *hypersensitivity* reaction to the injection of foreign *antigens* in large quantity especially those contained in *antisera* used for *passive immunization*. Symptoms appear some days after a single dose of the antigen (cf. *anaphylaxis*) and consist of local swelling at the injection site, enlarged *lymph nodes*, fever, *urticaria*, joint swellings and, more rarely, renal lesions. The symptoms are due to the localization in the tissues of soluble *immune complexes* (see *soluble complex*) formed between *antibody* produced during the developing *immune response*, and the large quantities of antigen still present. They take the form, therefore, of a generalized *Arthus reaction* (*type III hypersensitivity reaction*). See also *immune complex disease*.

severe combined immunodeficiency syndrome See *SCID*.

Sezary syndrome A *T cell*, *lymphoma* with erythroderma and other skin lesions. There are circulating T lymphoma cells with a characteristic irregular nuclear morphology. Associated with mycosis fungoides.

sheep cell agglutination test Any test in which sheep erythrocytes are *agglutinated* by *antibody* to them, or to material adsorbed to them as in the *Rose–Waaler test*.

short consensus repeat (SCR) A repeating domain of about 60 residues, found in proteins of the *SCR superfamily*.

Shwartzman reaction (Shwartzman–Sanarelli phenomenon) Local skin necrosis or generalized disease of kidneys, lungs, liver and heart following the second of two doses of *lipopolysaccharide* (LPS). Since LPS is a powerful inducer of inflammatory *cytokines* such as *TNF-α*, *IL-1* and others, these are likely to be implicated in its pathogenesis.

sIg Surface *immunoglobulin*. See *membrane immunoglobulin*. The prefix s is ambiguous and used for 'secretory' and 'soluble' etc., e.g. sIgA for *secretory IgA* found in external body secretions.

sIgA See *secretory IgA*.

signal hypothesis This is now the accepted explanation for the entry of the *heavy chains* and *light chains* of *immunoglobulins* into the *endoplasmic reticulum*, thus ensuring secretion of the assembled immunoglobulin molecules from the cell. The *leader peptide* of a nascent heavy or light chain, during synthesis on a ribosome, binds to a signal recognition particle (SRP) in the cytoplasm. The complex then binds to a SRP *receptor* in the membrane of the endoplasmic reticulum. The result is vectorial release of the heavy or light chain through the membrane into the cisternal space and secretion of the immunoglobulin after assembly of the polypeptide chains. The mechanism is common to most secreted proteins.

signal peptide See *leader peptide*.

Simonsen phenomenon A *graft-versus-host reaction*. Simonsen in 1957 observed splenomegaly in embryo chicks injected with *lymphocytes* derived from adult chickens. The embryo *spleens* contained increased numbers of lymphocytes partly derived from the donor, partly from the host.

single layer immunofluorescence technique See *direct immunofluorescence*.

single radial diffusion test A *quantitative gel diffusion test* in which one of the reactants (usually *antibody*) is incorporated into a layer of agar into which a well is then cut. The other reactant (usually *antigen*) is placed in the well and allowed to diffuse into the agar. A ring of precipitate (see *precipitation*) is formed, the area of which is proportional to the concentration of the material in the well. Usually used in the quantitative assay of antigens, especially *immunoglobulins*, incorporating a monospecific anti immunoglobulin serum in the agar. Frequently referred to as a Mancini test.

SJL mouse An *inbred strain* of mouse in which mature, but not young, animals develop a fatal autoimmune (see *autoimmunity*) haemolytic anaemia if injected with rat erythrocytes.

Sjögren's disease Chronic inflammatory disease of salivary and lachrymal glands in man often accompanied by secondary inflammation of the conjunctiva. In many cases, associated with *rheumatoid arthritis*. *Sera* of patients often contain *anti nuclear antibody* and *rheumatoid factor* as well as *antibody* against the duct epithelium of the salivary and lachrymal glands.

skin sensitizing antibody *IgE* antibody capable of attachment to skin *mast cells* so that, on subsequent combination with antigen, an *immediate hypersensitivity (type I hypersensitivity reaction), weal and flare response* occurs. At one time the presence of skin sensitizing IgE antibody in humans' serum was demonstrated by its intradermal transfer to a non-sensitized recipient; subsequent inoculation of the *allergen* produced a weal and flare (the PK test). An equivalent test in animals is *passive cutaneous anaphylaxis* (PCA).

skin test Any test in which substances are injected into or applied to the skin in order to observe the host's response to them. Used extensively in the investigation of *hypersensitivity* and *immunity* as in, e.g. the *tuberculin test*, etc.

skin window A technique employed to study the sequence of changes that occur in inflammation. The skin is scraped until capillary bleeding occurs. A small coverslip, or, better, a small chamber containing balanced salt solution is then applied and secured firmly in place. At intervals thereafter the cells which have migrated into the chamber are removed, stained, and identified.

SLE (systemic lupus erythematosus) Putative *autoimmune disease* of man, characterized by widespread focal degeneration, 'fibrinoid necrosis' of connective tissue and disseminated lesions in many tissues including skin, joints, kidneys, pleura, peripheral vessels, peripheral nervous system, blood etc. May follow administration of drugs or other *antigenic* substances. Numerous immunological abnormalities include presence in *serum* of *anti nuclear antibodies*, including *antibodies* to double-stranded DNA, antibodies to *ENAs*, high serum levels of *immunoglobulin*, and low levels of *C3* and *C4*. There is tissue damage due to deposition of *immune complexes*, especially of double-stranded DNA with anti DNA antibody. The glomerular lesions are particularly serious and have been shown to result from deposition of immune complexes in the glomerular capillaries. Cf. *lupus erythematosus*.

slot blotting See *dot blotting*.

slow reacting substance A (SRS-A) Name formerly used for vasoactive *leukotrienes* (LTC$_4$, D$_4$, and E$_4$).

small lymphocyte Cell 5–8 μm in diameter with a deeply staining nucleus and narrow rim of cytoplasm. The size simply indicates a resting (G0) cell and despite the apparent identity of morphology, small *lymphocytes* differ in origin and function. See *T lymphocyte, B lymphocyte*.

smallpox vaccination The classical *immunization* procedure introduced by Jenner who used *cowpox* virus, which cross reacts as an *antigen* with smallpox virus but is not pathogenic in man. The related *vaccinia* virus was used successfully for many years but *vaccination* against the disease has been abandoned since the elimination of smallpox worldwide.

soluble complex *Immune complex* in soluble form. Occurs *in vivo* or *in vitro* usually where there is an excess of *antigen* over *antibody* so that a lattice is not formed (see *lattice hypothesis*). Causes tissue damage *in vivo* (especially if *complement* is also bound); e.g. as soluble immune complexes easily become

trapped in small blood vessels this causes local aggregation of *neutrophil leucocytes* by *chemotaxis*, increase in vascular permeability, lodgement of neutrophils, fibrin, and *platelets* on vascular endothelium with oedema or thrombosis and necrosis. See *type III hypersensitivity reaction, Arthus reaction, serum sickness, glomerulonephritis, immune complex disease*.

somatic hypermutation Mutations that occur rapidly in the V-region (*variable region*) genes of the *light chain* and *heavy chain* during the formation of memory B cells (see *memory cells*), giving many more V-region sequences than are found in the germline genes from which they originated. The mutations are restricted to the V-regions only and the mutation rate has been estimated at approximately 10^{-3} per base pair per cell division. This is about 100 times the mutation rate in *pre-B lymphocytes* and proliferating cells in the secondary response. *Positive selection* follows interaction with *antigen* of those *B cells* that bear *membrane immunoglobulin* (*antibodies*) whose *affinity* has been increased by such mutations and, by ensuring survival of these B cells only, leads to an increase in the average affinity of the antibodies produced. Somatic hypermutation takes place in *germinal centres*.

Southern blotting A technique for the detection of DNA fragments containing defined sequences. After digestion with restriction enzymes, DNA fragments of different sizes are separated into bands by electrophoresis in Agarose® gel and transferred to a membrane by capillary blotting which produces an exact replica of the original pattern on the membrane. Bands of DNA containing defined sequences, e.g. a gene or *exon*, are detected by hybridization with radiolabelled cDNA. Widely used in molecular immunology. See also *northern blotting*.

SPA (staphylococcal protein A; SpA) See *protein A*.

specific granule Cytoplasmic granule of the *neutrophil leucocyte* containing *lysozyme*, lactoferrin, vitamin B_{12}-binding protein and neutral proteases. Smaller than the *azurophil granule* and probably appears later in development. Fuses more rapidly with *phagosomes* than the azurophil granule, and its contents are also readily secreted to the exterior.

specific immunity As a general concept, specific immunity is a non-susceptibility to re-infection by a pathogen, that develops in individuals who survive a first encounter with that same pathogen. The mechanisms which underlie this form of protection play a role in many aspects of bodily homeostasis other than defence against infection. 'Specific immunity' in this wider sense is: the *immunity²* resulting from *recognition* of *antigen* such that *antibody* and/or *T lymphocytes* are produced which can react specifically with that antigen.

specificity A term defining selective reactivity between substances, e.g. of an *antigen* with its corresponding *antibody* or *primed lymphocyte*.

spleen A solid, encapsulated organ, deep red in colour, found in the upper abdomen. It is a *peripheral lymphoid organ* which has a major arterial supply and acts as a blood filter. The spleen comprises two fundamentally distinct types of tissue, the 'white pulp' (Malpighian body or corpuscle) which is a *lymphoid tissue*, and the 'red pulp'. (a) The white pulp forms a cuff or sheath of tissue round the arterioles which consists chiefly of *lymphocytes* together with a smaller number of splenic *dendritic cells*. The central zone of the white pulp (nearest the arterioles) is a *thymus dependent area* and contains *T cells*. More peripherally are found *B cells* in spherical *lymphoid follicles*. *Germinal centres* (q.v.) develop in these follicles following *antigenic* stimulation. The arterioles terminate in venules between the white and the red pulp (the marginal zone) and it is from these venules that lymphocytes migrate into and populate the white pulp. The marginal zone itself is rich in B *memory cells* which are well placed to interact with antigens carried

in the blood. (b) The red pulp consists of large numbers of blood-filled sinusoids in which *phagocytosis* of effete erythrocytes takes place. It also functions as a reserve site for haemopoiesis. It is rich in *macrophages*, and *plasma cells* are also found there. See Figure S1.

splenectomy Surgical removal of the complete *spleen*. After splenectomy, the *immune response* to intravenously inoculated *antigens* is greatly reduced. Splenectomized subjects also show an increased susceptibility to septicaemia, e.g. with *Streptococcus pneumoniae*, and to blood-borne protozoal infections.

split tolerance (1) A result sometimes obtained following the experimental induction of *immunological tolerance* to *allogeneic* cells. Tolerance to one *antigen*, or to a group of antigens on the surfaces of those cells is produced, whilst simultaneously there is an active *immune response* to other antigens on the cells. (2) The term has also been used to refer to immunological tolerance affecting *either* **humoral immunity** or *cell-mediated immunity* but not both at the same time.

spur In *double diffusion tests* (especially *Ouchterlony tests*), a spur of precipitate (see *precipitation*) is indicative of a *reaction of partial identity* q.v.

SRBC Sheep erythrocytes (red blood cells).

SRS-A (slow reacting substance of anaphylaxis) Name formerly used for vasoactive *leukotrienes* (LTC_4, D_4, and E_4).

staphylococcal protein A See *protein A*.

stem cell The progenitor of all the cells of the immune system. A large cell with a rim of intensely RNA-rich (pyroninophilic, see *methyl green pyronin stain*) cytoplasm and pyroninophilic nucleoli within a leptochromatic nucleus (i.e. having narrow strands of chromatin) found in *bone marrow* and other haemopoietic tissues. Capable of both self-replication and generation of a

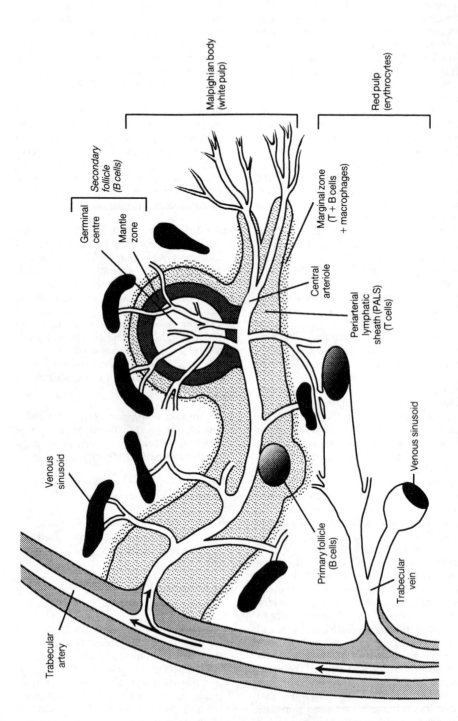

Figure S1. Spleen. Diagram of a section of a human spleen showing a Malpighian body containing a primary and secondary follicle with a germinal centre.

series of line-specific progenitor cells by proliferation and differentiation under the influence of *colony stimulating factors*. Known also as CFU-S (*colony forming unit*-spleen), referring to the tissue in which it was first studied.

streptococcal nephritis *Glomerulo-nephritis* following infection with *Streptococcus pyogenes* of Lancefield group A and, most commonly, of Griffith type 12. Associated with deposits containing *immunoglobulin* and *complement* in the glomeruli and probably reflects a *hypersensitivity* reaction (chiefly a *type III hypersensitivity reaction* due to *immune complexes*) either against streptococcal antigens deposited in the glomerulus itself or against a glomerular basement membrane antigen sharing *epitopes* with the streptococcus (in this case a response of *autoimmunity*). Nephritis has been produced after injection of animals with streptococcal antigens but it differs from the human disease in many respects.

stromal cells See *reticular cells*.

subset Term used to classify functionally or structurally different populations of cells within a single cell type.

subunit vaccines *Vaccines* which are part of a pathogen. These are either randomly broken down materials, or chemically purified and defined materials from whole organisms. Some subunit vaccines are produced by recombinant DNA techniques (see *recombinant vaccine*).

superantigen Designation of a class of *antigen* that activates all *T cells* bearing a particular *TCR* Vβ sequence. Superantigens are presented on *class II MHC antigens*, but do not require to be processed and do not bind as peptides in the groove of the class II molecule. Thus presentation is not *MHC restricted* and *recognition* is not limited to individual clones of *T lymphocytes*. Superantigens bind with high *affinity* to a region of class II MHC molecules that is outside the groove and to a region of the TCR Vβ chain away from the *antigen-binding site*, forming a direct link between MHC

and TCR. Many superantigens are of microbial origin, e.g. staphylococcal enterotoxins, toxic shock syndrome toxin, streptococcal exotoxin A, *Mycoplasma arthritidis* mitogen. *Mls* antigens (q.v.) are self-superantigens.

superfamily A group of proteins which show structural homology and putatively evolved from the same primordial gene.

superoxide anion (O_2^-) Oxygen molecule that carries an extra unpaired electron, and is therefore a free radical. Generated in *neutrophil leucocytes* and *mononuclear phagocytes* by one-electron-step reduction of molecular oxygen, by an NADPH oxidase (cytochrome b), driven by hexose monophosphate shunt pathway activation. Highly reactive and toxic O_2^- may be further reduced to H_2O_2, or, when two O_2^- radicals interact, one is oxidized and the other reduced in a dismutation reaction to form O_2 and H_2O_2. This reaction is catalysed by superoxide dismutase, an enzyme present in *phagocytic* cells. O_2^-, H_2O_2 and the hydroxyl radical OH play a major part in the oxidative microbicidal activity of neutrophils and mononuclear phagocytes (see also *myeloperoxidase*).

suppressor T lymphocyte Presently ill-defined subpopulation of *T lymphocytes* which directly suppresses the *immune response*.

surface immunoglobulin See *membrane immunoglobulin*.

surrogate light chain A protein found in precursors of *B cells* (*pro-B lymphocytes* and *pre-B lymphocytes*) but not in mature B lymphocytes. Derived from the genes $V_{pre\ B}$ and λ_5 which do not undergo *translocation* (see *immunoglobulin gene*) but are transcribed separately. The $V_{pre\ B}$ and λ_5 polypeptides form *light chain*-like structures which associate with the μ *heavy chain* (of *IgM*) made by B cell precursors before they start to make functional light chains.

switch region The region of DNA 5′ to each *heavy chain* C-region gene containing the *switch sites* q.v.

switch site A short sequence of DNA 5' to each *heavy chain* C-region gene but not continuous with it, which acts as a recognition site for *translocation* of the VDJ exon during switching of gene expression from one *heavy chain class* to another (see *isotype switching*). Each C-region gene has multiple switch sites contained within the *switch region*.

sympathetic ophthalmia Inflammatory disease of a sound eye following perforating injury of the other eye. Characterized by *lymphocyte* and *epithelioid cell* infiltration and *granuloma* formation, especially in the uveal tract. Postulated reaction of *cell-mediated immunity* against *antigens*, normally *sequestered antigens*, liberated by injury to the opposite eye, thus an *auto-immune disease*.

syngeneic (syngenic) Genetically identical, usually applied to grafts made within an *inbred strain*. See also *transplantation terminology*.

synthetic peptide vaccine *Vaccines* based on oligopeptides synthesized chemically. They are normally 15–25 residues long, corresponding to regions of protein macromolecules which have been identified to be highly *immunogenic* and can induce *protective immunity* against targeted pathogens. These vaccines are precisely defined, easy to produce and do not need to be stored under refrigeration, thus easing distribution. However, they are likely to be weakly immunogenic and may be genetically restricted in their ability to activate *T cells*.

systemic anaphylaxis See *anaphylaxis*.

systemic lupus erythematosus See *SLE*.

T

T–B cell cooperation A process required for production of normal levels of *antibody* to *thymus dependent antigens*, i.e. most *antigens*. Requires physical contact of *helper T lymphocytes* and *B lymphocytes* with *accessory cells*.

T cell See *T lymphocyte*; the two names are interchangeable.

T cell-dependent antigen See *thymus dependent antigen*.

T cell-dependent area See *thymus dependent area*.

T cell-dependent immune response The *immune response* of *cell-mediated immunity*. The latter term was introduced before *T cells* were discovered and is inexact but universally used.

T cell receptor See *TCR*.

T cell subset See *T lymphocyte subset*.

T cell tyrosine kinase See *protein tyrosine kinase*.

T-dependent antigen See *thymus dependent antigen*.

T-dependent area See *thymus dependent area*.

T helper cell See *helper T lymphocyte*.

T-independent antigen See *thymus independent antigen*.

T lymphocyte (also called a T cell; the two names are interchangeable) *Lymphocyte* that is derived from the *thymus*. Carries an *antigen*-specific *T cell receptor*, and is *CD3+*. T lymphocytes play a major role (a) as antigen reactive cells and effector cells in *cell-mediated immunity*; and (b) by cooperating with

B lymphocytes, in *antibody* production (*humoral immunity*) against *thymus dependent antigens*.

T lymphocyte antigen receptor See *TCR*.

T lymphocyte–B lymphocyte cooperation See *T–B cell cooperation*.

T lymphocyte repertoire The number of different *epitopes* to which the *T lymphocytes* of an individual animal are capable of responding. Cf. *B lymphocyte repertoire* and see *repertoire*.

T lymphocyte subset Group of *T lymphocytes* which are identified phenotypically by specific cell surface antigens and are characterized by a particular function. See *helper T lymphocyte, cytotoxic T lymphocyte, T_{DTH} lymphocyte* and *CD antigens*.

T lymphocyte–T lymphocyte cooperation Postulated interaction between different *T lymphocyte subsets* in activation of *cell-mediated immune responses*. See also *T–B cell cooperation*.

T zone See *thymus dependent area*.

T6 marker Mouse chromosome originally derived from an irradiated male. It is about half the length of the shortest pair of autosomes, and has a marked secondary constriction near the centromere. It is a useful cell marker, easily identifiable in squash preparations of somatic tissues and can therefore be used for tracing the fate of cells transferred to another mouse. Present in the *inbred strain* CBA/H-T6.

tachyphylaxis Reduction in responsiveness of cells or tissues to a stimulus, induced as a result of prior exposure to the same or a related stimulus.

tail peptide A polypeptide at the C-terminus of a *heavy chain* which is not a part of the C-terminal domain. The secreted forms of *IgA* and *IgM* have tail peptides (T$_s$) 20 amino acids long, not found in *IgG* or *IgE*. The membrane forms of all immunoglobulins (see *membrane immunoglobulin*) have predominantly hydrophobic tail peptides (T$_m$) different from the secreted form. The T$_m$ of the μ_m chain is 41 amino acids long, that of the γ_m chain is approximately 70 amino acids long.

tanned red cell test A sensitive *passive agglutination test* for the detection and measurement of *antibody*. Treatment of erythrocytes with tannic acid increases their agglutinability and facilitates the attachment ('coating') to them of soluble proteins.

TAP (transporter associated with antigen processing) Proteins derived from *MHC gene*-associated *Tap* genes. TAP proteins transport the peptides generated from cytoplasmic cleavage of endogenously synthesized proteins across the membrane into the lumen of the *endoplasmic reticulum*, where they associate with, and stabilize, *class I MHC antigen* molecules. TAP proteins are essential for presentation (see *antigen presentation*)

of *antigen* with class I MHC. See Figure A2.

TCR (T cell receptor; T lymphocyte receptor; TcR) The molecule on the surface membrane of *T lymphocytes* capable of specifically binding *antigen* in association with *MHC* antigens. The molecule belongs to the *Ig superfamily* and consists of two *Type I transmembrane protein* disulphide-linked polypeptide chains of molecular weight 40–50 kD. The majority (~90%) of human T lymphocytes express a TCR composed of an $\alpha\beta$ heterodimer, while the remaining, mutually exclusive, population of T cells expresses a $\gamma\delta$ TCR. Each chain contains a variable (V) and constant (C) region, homologous to those found in *immunoglobulin* molecule *variable regions* and *constant regions*. In addition, the β and δ chains contain junctional (J) and diversity (D) regions which are analogous to those in immunoglobulin molecules. The α and γ chains also contain junctional regions. The *antigen-binding site* is formed primarily from the combination of the D and J regions with a small contribution from the V region and is responsible for interacting both with foreign peptide and self MHC molecules. The TCR is always non-covalently linked in the T

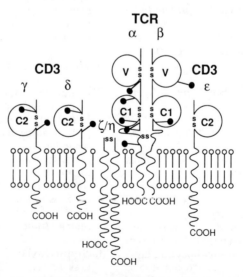

Figure T1. TCR. Diagram of a TCR/CD3 complex and associated polypeptide chains in the lipid bilayer of a T cell membrane. ↑, N-linked glycosylation site.

cell membrane to the **CD3** molecule, q.v. See Figure T1.

TCR genes See Figure T2.

TD antigen See *thymus dependent antigen*.

TdT (terminal deoxynucleotidyl transferase) An enzyme found in *pre-B lymphocytes* and cortical *thymocytes* (see *thymus*) but absent from their progeny. It is responsible for the random addition of nucleotides at the 5′ end of the *D exon* (the N region) during V–D gene recombination, thus increasing the diversity of the *antigen-binding site*. This process occurs in both *heavy chains* of *immunoglobulins* and α, β, γ and δ chains of the *TCR*.

T$_{DTH}$ lymphocyte Effector *T lymphocyte* in *delayed-type hypersensitivity* reaction. Usually *CD4*+ and putatively may belong to the *T$_H$1* subset of CD4+ cells. Function depends on production of *cytokines* such as *IFN-γ*.

terminal deoxynucleotidyl transferase See *TdT*.

test dosing A hazardous technique used to detect *immediate hypersensitivity* to drugs or *antisera* before a therapeutic dose is given. Ideally, doses that increase by tenfold steps are given daily until a reaction occurs or a therapeutic level is reached, the starting point being at the microgram level for orally administered materials, and at nanogram level for those given parenterally. *Skin testing* (q.v.) is usually preferable but even this is potentially hazardous. Corticosteroid and adrenalin cover is often required in these procedures. See also *hyposensitization*.

tetramethylrhodamine isothiocyanate A red fluorescent dye (see *fluorochrome*) which combines with protein in alkaline solution. Used in *immunofluorescence* techniques.

tetraparental chimera A *chimera* (usually mouse) resulting from the artificially induced fusion of two blastocysts at the 4 or 8 cell stage. Of immunological importance as demonstrates maintenance of mutual *immunological tolerance*.

TGF-β (transforming growth factor β$_{1-5}$) A family of protein *cytokines* derived from *lymphocytes*, *macrophages* and other tissue cells. Exhibit a wide range of pleiotropic effects, including inhibition of cell turnover, induction of differentiation and stimulation of collagen production. Important immunological effects include *immunosuppression*, regulation of *T lymphocyte* differentiation, wound healing, induction of integrin (see *integrin superfamily*) expression and class-specific *isotype switching* in *B lymphocytes* to *IgA*.

T$_H$ lymphocyte *Helper T lymphocyte*. See *T$_H$1 cells* and *T$_H$2 cells*.

T$_H$1 cells Functional *T lymphocyte subset* of *CD4*+ cells, characterized by their

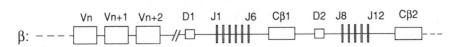

Figure T2. Mouse TCR gene loci. There are 13 families of Vα exons with 3–20 members in each, giving 50–100 Vα exons in total and 75–100 Vβ exons, approximately 50 Jα and 12 functional Jβ. The human α and β gene loci are broadly similar to mouse. The δ gene locus is between the last Vα and Jα1. The γ gene locus has two families of J exons and two C exons, similar to the β chain.

production of the *cytokines IL-2, IFN-γ* and *TNF-α, -β* and by failure to produce *IL-4, IL-5* and *IL-10*. A polarization of the immune response towards T$_H$1 cell activity can occur in mice (and possibly man) and is associated with *cell-mediated immunity in vivo* including *delayed-type hypersensitivity* and T cell proliferation. The selective activation of T$_H$1 cells is favoured by the presence of IFN-γ and *IL-12* and is inhibited by IL-4 and IL-10 (cf. *T$_H$2 cells*).

T$_H$2 cells Functional *T lymphocyte subset* of *CD4+* cells which, in mice (and possibly man) is distinct from the *T$_H$1 subset*, q.v. T$_H$2 cells are characterized by the production of *IL-4, IL-5* and *IL-10* and by the failure to produce *IL-2* and *IFN-γ*. T$_H$2 cell activation is associated with helper activity for antibody production (see *helper T lymphocyte*) and the inhibition of T$_H$1-mediated responses. IL-4 is essential for the growth and differentiation of T$_H$2 cells.

thoracic duct drainage Surgical technique used in man and in experimental animals whereby circulating *lymphocytes* (see *lymphocyte recirculation*) can be withdrawn through a catheter inserted into the thoracic duct.

Thy 1 (CDw90; previously known as theta (θ) antigen) A small *GPI anchor*-linked protein of the *Ig superfamily* with a single *variable region* (V)-like domain. Marker of *thymus*-derived *lymphocytes* in the mouse, being present on *thymocytes* as well as on *T lymphocytes* in the *peripheral lymphoid organs*. It is also present in central nervous tissue. In humans, found on early thymocytes and in the central nervous system. See Figure T3.

thymectomy Surgical removal of the *thymus*. If carried out immediately after birth (neonatal thymectomy) a deficiency of *cell-mediated immunity* and of *humoral immunity* to *thymus dependent antigens* follows. See also *wasting disease*.

thymic cortex See *thymus*.

thymic epithelial cells Epithelial cells found in the thymic cortex and medulla

(see *thymus*) and derived from the third branchial pouch. They are believed to control the *education* of *T lymphocyte* precursors by presenting self-peptides bound to MHC (*major histocompatibility complex*) molecules and by secreting *cytokines* which stimulate *lymphocyte* growth.

thymic hypoplasia Congenital *cell-mediated immunity* deficiency syndrome in human infants. Often associated with hypoparathyroidism (see *Di George's syndrome*). The blood *lymphocyte* count is low, *T lymphocytes* being completely absent and the *thymus dependent areas* of *lymphoid tissues* are depleted of lymphocytes. T-dependent *B lymphocyte* responses are also impaired. Recurrent opportunistic infections of the skin and respiratory tract may be present.

thymic medullary hyperplasia Term used to signify the presence of *germinal centres* in the medulla of the *thymus* especially in *myasthenia gravis*. The term does not imply that thymic weight is increased. The situation has been confused by the identification of germinal centres in thymuses of normal subjects.

thymic nurse cell Large thymic epithelial cell (see *thymus*) with which *thymocytes* come into close contact. Postulated role in maturation and differentiation of *T lymphocytes*.

thymocyte Any *lymphocyte* found within the *thymus*.

thymus The organ essential for the development of *T lymphocytes*. In mammals it consists of two lobes situated in the anterior part of the thorax, ventral to the trachea and great vessels and is derived from the third and fourth branchial pouches. In birds, it is distributed along the neck as a series of lobes. Histologically, it consists mainly of *lymphocytes* distributed into distinct cortical and medullary areas on a network of *reticular cells* (stromal cells). In the cortex, these lymphocytes ('thymocytes') are rapidly dividing progeny of T lymphocyte precursors derived from haemopoietic tissues. During development in the cortex thymocytes are initially *CD4–CD8–*, but then become CD4+CD8+ and eventually develop into either CD4+CD8– or CD4–CD8+, at which point they accumulate in the medulla before leaving to populate the *peripheral lymphoid organs* as mature T cells. CD4–CD8–thymocytes begin to rearrange T cell receptor (*TCR*) genes randomly and, depending on the surface receptor expressed, undergo *positive selection* and *negative selection*. As a result, 95% of the thymocytes produced never leave the thymus and die. In addition to lymphocytes the thymus contains large numbers of epithelial cells, stromal cells and accessory *dendritic cells* which play important roles in positive and negative selection, both by presentation of self MHC (*major histocompatibility complex*) molecules and by production of growth factors for lymphocytes. The thymus functions mainly in the fetal and early neonatal period, and animals *thymectomized* at birth or congenitally athymic (see *nude mice, thymic hypoplasia*) have an absence of T lymphocytes. After puberty, the thymus atrophies, but may continue to produce new T lymphocytes and animals thymectomized during adult life gradually become deficient in T cells.

thymus dependent antigen (T-dependent antigen) An *antigen* that does not stimulate an *antibody* response in animals lacking a *thymus*. Cooperation with *helper T lymphocytes* is required in order for *B lymphocytes* to respond to such antigens by maturation into antibody-forming cells. Most proteins and other antigens which present a diversity of *epitopes* are thymus dependent. Cf. *thymus independent antigens.*

thymus dependent area Those areas of the *peripheral lymphoid organs* that appear selectively depleted of *lymphocytes* in neonatally *thymectomized* animals, and in babies and animals with congenital aplasia of the *thymus* (see *thymic hypoplasia* and *nude* mice). Anatomically these areas are situated in the mid cortex (paracortical area) of *lymph nodes*, the centre of the Malpighian corpuscle of the *spleen* and in the internodular zone of *Peyer's patches*. In normal subjects they are mostly occupied by *small lymphocytes* of the recirculatory pool (see *lymphocyte recirculation*) which enter them by crossing *high endothelial venules*. They also contain various *accessory cells* including *macrophages* and *dendritic cells* (*interdigitating cells*). See Figure L1.

thymus dependent cells Population of *lymphocytes* whose normal development depends on the presence of the *thymus* at birth, i.e. *T lymphocytes* q.v.

thymus derived cells *T lymphocytes*. Most T lymphocytes, but perhaps not all, require to mature in the *thymus*.

thymus independent antigen (T-independent antigen) An *antigen* that is able to stimulate *B lymphocytes* to produce *antibody* without the cooperation of *T lymphocytes*. An antibody response to such antigens can be stimulated in an animal lacking a *thymus*. T-independent antigens are, frequently, repeating polymers which present an array of identical *epitopes* to the lymphocyte; see *TI-1 antigen* and *TI-2 antigen*. Cf. *thymus dependent antigen.*

thymus independent antigen Type 1 See *TI-1 antigen.*

thymus independent antigen Type 2 See *TI-2 antigen.*

thyroid antibodies Organ-specific *autoantibodies* found in a variety of thyroid diseases, especially *Hashimoto's thyroiditis* and *thyrotoxicosis*. The major *antibodies* are those against thyroglobulin, against thyroid peroxidase and against thyroid stimulating hormone (TSH) receptors which mimic the action of TSH.

thyroiditis Inflammatory disease of the thyroid gland. Rarely due to bacterial infection, but de Quervain's thyroiditis is probably due to mumps virus. Riedel's thyroiditis is a slow fibrous replacement of unknown cause. *Hashimoto's thyroiditis*, primary hypothyroidism (myxoedema), and chronic focal thyroiditis may result from *autoimmunity*.

See also *thyrotoxicosis, thyroid antibodies*.

thyrotoxicosis   *Autoimmune* disease characterized by increase in level of circulating thyroid hormones usually associated with hyperplasia or hypertrophy of the thyroid gland, either diffuse or nodular, with *lymphocyte* infiltration, and circulating *autoantibodies* against thyroid *antigens*. The major *antibody* is directed against the *receptors* for thyroid stimulating hormone (TSH), and stimulates thyroid function by binding to these receptors.

TI-1 antigen   (thymus independent antigen Type 1) An *antigen* which activates *B cells* in the absence of *T cell* help (see *helper T lymphocyte*) by by-passing the normal signalling pathway through the antigen *receptor*. These molecules, e.g. bacterial *lipopolysaccharides* (LPS) or poly I:poly C, are usually *polyclonal activators* at high concentrations since they bind to *mitogen* receptor molecules on the surface of most B cells and activate the cell independently of the specific antigen receptor. At low concentrations they bind only to B cells with specific antigen receptors and the resulting concentration of the TI-1 antigen on the B cell surface results in activation of the B cell through the mitogen receptor pathway.

TI-2 antigen   (thymus independent antigen Type 2) Multivalent *antigens*, often polysaccharides, containing repeating *epitopes*, which activate a subpopulation of *B lymphocytes* in the absence of *T cell* help. They persist for long periods in *macrophages* and, unlike *TI-1 antigens*, activate the B cell by cross linking the antigen *receptor*. Examples include *pneumococcal polysaccharide*, dextran sulphate (see *dextrans*), TNP (trinitrophenylated)-Ficoll® and polymerized *flagellin*. In some cases these antigens selectively activate *B-1 lymphocytes*.

tingible body macrophage   *Macrophage* within a *germinal centre* that has phagocytosed apoptotic (see *apoptosis*) *B lymphocytes*. The 'tingible bodies' (deeply staining debris) are remnants of ingested cells.

tissue specific antigen   Cell *antigen* present in a given tissue and not found in other tissues, e.g. thyroglobulin is tissue specific for the thyroid. Important in classification of *autoimmune diseases* in which *autoantibodies* against either tissue specific antigens or non-tissue specific antigens are found. These antigens are often not species specific, e.g. anti human thyroglobulin reacts with thyroglobulin from many other species.

tissue typing   See *histocompatibility testing*.

titre   (USA titer) A measure of the activity of a reagent obtained by *serial dilution* of the reactants and often expressed in arbitrary units as an end point dilution. Has been used widely for measuring the quantity of *antibody* in *antisera*, but has much wider applications.

Tla antigen   Murine class III MHC antigen (see *H-2 histocompatibility system*), coded for by genes located on chromosome 17 distal to the *H-2D/H-2L* region. Recognized, by specific *alloantisera*, with as many as six possible allelic products, on *thymocytes*. This region is closely associated with the *Qa* region (see *Qa antigens*). Tl antigens appear anomalously on leukaemia cells.

T_m C-terminal polypeptide (*tail peptide*, q.v.) of the *heavy chain* of *membrane immunoglobulin*. Associated in the cell membrane with *CD79*a and b.

TM4 superfamily   (transmembrane 4 pass superfamily) A group of *Type III transmembrane proteins* which traverse the membrane bilayer four times. Includes the β chain of FcεRI (see *Fcε receptors*). See Figure T3.

TNF   (tumour necrosis factor) Note that *TNF-α* and *TNF-β* (below) are also frequently called TNF and LT (lymphotoxin) respectively. Thus, in many publications the designation TNF, without a following Greek letter, refers to the *cytokine*, TNF-α.

TNF-α (tumour necrosis factor α; also known as cachectin) A *cytokine* of MW 17 kD which normally exists as a trimer. The name 'tumour necrosis factor' derives from early observations that this cytokine could kill tumour cells in tissue culture and, presumptively, *in vivo*. TNF-α is made by *mononuclear phagocytes, neutrophil leucocytes, NK cells, activated lymphocytes*, activated vascular endothelial cells and others and has a gene close to, and shares some structural homology and many functions with, *TNF-β*, made by *lymphocytes*. TNF-α has an extremely wide range of activity; it is a prominent inflammatory cytokine whose release by *macrophages* is activated by *lipopolysaccharide* (LPS) and other bacterial products. Like *IL-1*, it is a pyrogen, induces *leucocytosis*, enhances endothelial adhesiveness, is a primer of neutrophil function, enhances production of other cytokines and of *acute phase reactants*, *inter alia*. Overproduction of TNF-α is associated with *septic shock* induced by LPS and other bacterial products, and with wasting (cachexia: hence the name cachectin) in patients with neoplasia or infectious disease.

TNF-β (tumour necrosis factor β; lymphotoxin; LT; LT-α) A *cytokine* of MW 25 kD (monomer) which normally exists as a trimer and shares some sequence homology but many functions with *TNF-α*. It is synthesized by *antigen*-activated or *mitogen*-activated *lymphocytes*, and has cytolytic activity for tumour cells and non-tumour cell lines in culture, hence the name, 'lymphotoxin'. It may be important for the activity of *cytotoxic T lymphocytes*. It binds to the same *receptors* as TNF-α and may share its pro-inflammatory properties.

TNF family A group of related proteins all of which usually exist as trimers and which bind to members of the *TNFR superfamily*. The family includes *TNF-α* and *TNF-β* (*LT*) (both of which bind to *TNFR-I and II*), LT-β (see LT; which binds to LT), Fas ligand (which binds to *Fas*), *CD40L* (which binds to *CD40*) and CD70 (which binds to CD27).

TNFR I and II (CD120a and b) *Type I transmembrane proteins* that are *recep-tors* for *TNF-α* and *TNF-β* and are present on almost all cell types. They belong to the *TNFR superfamily*. Both types of TNF bind as trimers to both receptors with high *affinity*. TNFR I is a 55 kD protein which mediates the lytic activity of TNF-α, while TNFR II (75 kD) mediates proliferative and regulatory signals. Soluble TNFR is found in biological fluids and may be important for neutralizing TNF activity. The TNFRs co-modulate (see *modulation*) with *Fas* (also a member of the TNFR family), an important mediator of *apoptosis*.

TNFR superfamily (tumour necrosis factor receptor superfamily) A family of molecules named the TNFR superfamily by immunologists and the NGFR (nerve growth factor receptor) superfamily by others. As well as *TNFR I and II*, and NGFR, other molecules in this superfamily are CD27 (which binds CD70), CD30 (which binds CD30 *ligand*), *CD40* (which binds *CD40L*) and *Fas* (which binds Fas ligand), all trimeric members of the *TNF family*. Binding of these trimers to their *receptors* may induce the latter also to form trimers which may be important for signal transduction.

tolerance See *immunological tolerance*.

tolerogenic Capable of inducing *immunological tolerance*.

tonsil Accumulations of *lymphoid tissue* found in invaginations of the mucous membrane in the area between the mouth and the pharynx. Tonsils vary in extent in different species being extensive in man and the horse, and small in cattle. They are not found in mice. In man they form distinct organs. The most prominent of these are the two palatine tonsils; tubal, lingual and a single nasopharyngeal tonsil complete a ring round the area. The tonsil is a *peripheral lymphoid organ*. It contains a high proportion of *B lymphocytes* and is almost always rich in *germinal centres*. Tonsillar tissue is widely used for the study of B lymphocyte function. In birds, aggregations of lymphoid tissue with germinal centres found in each caecal wall near the point at which the twin caeca enter the junction of the large and small intestines are called 'caecal tonsils'.

toxoid Bacterial *exotoxin* (e.g. diphtheria or tetanus toxin) which has been treated, usually with formalin, so that its ability to stimulate the production of *protective immunity* remains but it is no longer toxic and can therefore safely be used for *immunization*.

transfection The artificial transfer of foreign DNA into a eukaryotic cell.

transformation See *lymphocyte activation*.

transfusion reaction Disease or physiological disturbance following transfusion of blood. Often due to a specific immune reaction of the recipient against *antigens* on the donor's red blood cells. In man the most common and severe form of such reactions is due to *ABO blood group system* (q.v.) incompatibility as the recipient's plasma contains *natural antibodies* against the ABO antigens not present on his own cells. After repeated transfusions antibodies may be formed against other antigens on donor cells and cause reactions.

transgene A gene that has been *transfected* into the germ line to form a transgenic organism, e.g. a *transgenic mouse*.

transgenic mouse A mouse that carries a *transgene* that can be passed on to succeeding generations. The gene (DNA) is microinjected into fertilized eggs which are allowed to develop *in utero*. If the gene has been introduced into the germ line, the mice, as adults, will pass it on to their offspring. The mice that develop from *transfected* eggs are screened for the gene and selected mice are bred to achieve stable transmission of the gene.

translocation The movement of a gene or *exon* from its original site in the DNA to a new position on the same chromosome, e.g. the *V exons* and *D exons* of *immunoglobulin genes* and of the T cell receptor (*TCR*) move from their original position in the germline DNA to a new position adjacent to one of the *J exons* (hence the name 'joining') during differ-

entiation of a *stem cell* to a *B lymphocyte* or *T lymphocyte*. The J exon does not move. See Figures I4 and I5.

transplantation antigen See *histocompatibility antigen*.

transplantation immunology The study of the *immune response* following transplantation of tissue from donor to recipient. Very largely, the study of *cell-mediated immunity* in this situation.

transplantation terminology See Table T1.

transport piece See *secretory piece*.

trypan blue Stain used to assess the viability of cells. Cells whose membrane permeability is normal do not take up trypan blue but when the plasma membrane is severely disrupted, it allows the dye in. Dead and dying cells may therefore stain blue, but not if they die by *apoptosis* in which case membrane permeability may not be affected.

T_s C-terminal polypeptide (*tail peptide*, q.v.) of the *heavy chain* of secreted *immunoglobulin* continuing beyond the C-terminal domain, as in *IgA* and *IgM*.

tuberculin The crude protein extract from *Mycobacterium tuberculosis* from which *PPD* (q.v.) is derived.

tuberculin test Test for *delayed-type hypersensitivity* to *tuberculin* in man or animals. In man carried out by intradermal injection of *PPD*, see *Mantoux test*. Positive reactions are presumptive evidence of *cell-mediated immunity* to, and therefore of past or present exposure to, *Mycobacterium tuberculosis* but are in no sense diagnostic of active disease.

tumour necrosis factor α See *TNF-α*.

tumour necrosis factor β See *TNF-β*.

tumour specific antigen *Antigen* gained by any given tumour (see *antigen gain*). Tumour antigens may be: (a) identical to antigens present in parent tissues (and therefore in no sense tumour specific); (b) not present in par-

Table T1. Transplantation terminology

Present nomenclature	Older nomenclature	Relationship of donor and recipient of graft
Syngeneic (*isogeneic*) graft	*Autograft*	Same individual
Syngeneic (*isogeneic*) graft	*Homograft*	Same species and genetically identical
Allogeneic graft	Homograft	Same species but not genetically identical
Xenogeneic graft	Heterograft	Different species

ent tissue but found in other unrelated normal tissues; (c) fetal antigens not normally expressed in the adult, e.g. carcinoembryonic antigen; or (d) unique to the tumour. Experimental tumours induced by any given virus all bear identical tumour specific antigens, probably coded for by viral nuclear material incorporated into the host cell genome. However, the antigens in tumours induced by chemical carcinogens are different in each animal and even in multiple tumours in the same animal.

type I hypersensitivity reaction Term used in Gell and Coombs' classification of *hypersensitivity* reactions. In the type I reaction, *antigen* combines with *antibody* which is fixed passively to the surfaces of cells, usually *mast cells*, and causes the release of vasoactive substances, thus synonymous with *immediate hypersensitivity* and *anaphylaxis*. The cell bound antibody involved is usually *IgE*; the antigen is often known as an *allergen*. Typical diseases are *hay fever* and *asthma*.

type II hypersensitivity reaction Term used in Gell and Coombs' classification of *hypersensitivity* reactions. In the type II reaction, *antibody* reacts either with a cell surface *antigen* or with an antigen or *hapten* which has become attached to the cell surface. Typical diseases include *Goodpasture's syndrome* and *transfusion reactions*. If the antibody is *complement fixing antibody*, cell lysis occurs. See also *immune cytolysis*.

type III hypersensitivity reaction Term used in Gell and Coombs' classi-

fication of *hypersensitivity* reactions. In this reaction the tissue damage is mediated by *immune complexes*, particularly *soluble complexes* formed in slight *antigen excess*. Typical diseases include *serum sickness*, *extrinsic allergic alveolitis* and systemic lupus erythematosus (*SLE*). In such diseases the complexes are deposited in the blood vessel walls and become surrounded by *inflammatory cells*, especially *neutrophil leucocytes* in the acute phase. Later these are replaced by a *mononuclear cell* infiltrate. See also *Arthus reaction* and *glomerulonephritis*.

type IV hypersensitivity reaction Term used in Gell and Coombs' classification of *hypersensitivity* reactions. In the type IV reaction, *primed lymphocytes* react with *antigen* at the site of its deposition resulting in the formation of a *lymphocyte–macrophage granuloma*, e.g. in pulmonary tuberculosis. Circulating *antibody* is not involved in this reaction. See *delayed-type hypersensitivity* and *cell-mediated immunity*.

Type I transmembrane protein A membrane protein in which the N-terminal region is extracellular, there is a single hydrophobic membrane-spanning region, and the C-terminal region is intracytoplasmic. A large majority of membrane-spanning proteins are of this type. See Figure T3.

Type II transmembrane protein A membrane protein in which the C-terminal region is extracellular, there is a single hydrophobic membrane-spanning region, and the N-terminal

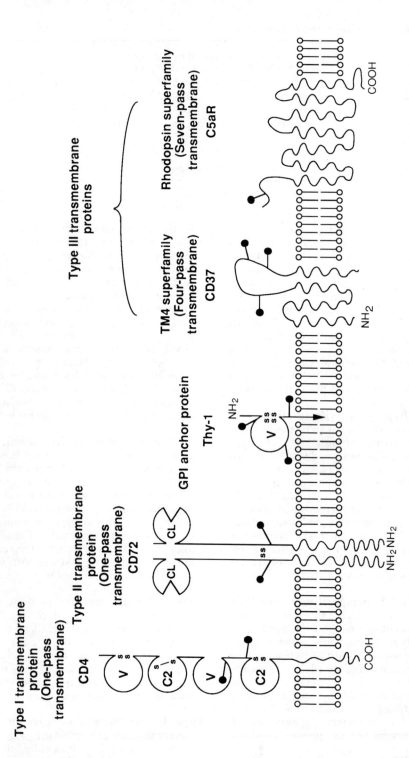

Figure T3. Transmembrane proteins. An illustration of the different ways in which membrane proteins are held in the lipid bilayer of the plasma membrane. The positions of N-linked (|) and O-linked (/) glycosylation sites are indicated.

region is intracytoplasmic. See Figure T3.

Type III transmembrane protein A membrane protein which is folded so that the molecule crosses the membrane more than once. An important group which does this is the *rhodopsin superfamily* containing the *chemotaxis* receptors for *formyl peptides*, *C5a* and the *chemokine* family. These have seven membrane-spanning domains and their N-terminal regions are outside, and the C-terminal regions inside, the cell. Another group, with four membrane-spanning domains (the *TM4 superfamily*), has both N- and C-termini within the cytoplasm. The β chain of the high *affinity* receptor for *IgE* (FcεRI, see *Fcε receptors*) is of this type. See Figure T3.

tyrosine kinase See *protein tyrosine kinase*.

U

ulcerative colitis Disease of man characterized by ulceration of the rectum and colon with diarrhoea and blood and mucus in the stools. Intermittent course, with considerable variation in the severity of symptoms and extent of colon involved. High incidence of carcinoma of the colon. Patients' *lymphocytes* may show cytotoxicity for colon epithelial cells and an *immune response* to mucosal *antigens* has been postulated as an aetiological factor. The mucosal inflammation is also associated with production of *cytokines* such as *IL-1*.

univalent antibody *Antibody* molecule with only a single *antigen-binding site*, therefore reacting with only one molecule of *antigen* and unable to form antigen–antibody precipitates but capable of 'blocking' *precipitation* of antigen by divalent antibodies. Separated *Fab fragments* obtained by *papain hydrolysis* have only one antigen-binding site and therefore behave in this way.

unprimed Having never had contact with or responded to a given *antigen* (of animals, cells, etc.). The terms 'naive' and 'virgin' are also used to describe unprimed *lymphocytes*.

unresponsiveness See *immunological unresponsiveness*.

uropod Elongated tail of a cell in locomotion. Term used especially of *lymphocytes* but applicable to all *leucocytes*. Moving lymphocytes sometimes show a 'hand mirror' appearance in which the uropod resembles the handle of the mirror.

urticaria (hives) Skin rash characterized by localized, elevated, erythematous, itchy weals due to local release of *histamine* and other vasoactive substances. Frequently associated with *immediate hypersensitivity* (*type I hypersensitivity reaction*) on contact of the skin with *allergens*, or more generalized as in *food allergy*.

V

V exon Gene coding for the *variable region* of the *heavy chain* or *light chain* of *immunoglobulins* and the α, β, γ and δ chains of the *TCR*. There are many different V exons in germline DNA, separated by a large region of untranslated DNA from the *D exon*, *J exon* and *C exon*, but in *B lymphocytes* and *T lymphocytes* one V exon has been translocated to a position adjacent to a J exon (Ig$_L$ locus) or a D exon (Ig$_H$ and T cell receptor loci). See Figures I5 and T2.

V-gene See *V exon*.

V-region See *variable region*.

vaccination Production of *active immunity* (*protective immunity*) in man or animal by administration of *vaccines*. An extension, by Louis Pasteur, of the original use of the word by Edward Jenner to describe the use of *cowpox* to protect against smallpox (*variola*, see *smallpox vaccination*).

vaccine A prophylactic or therapeutic material containing *antigens* derived from one or more pathogenic organisms which, on administration to man or animal, will stimulate *active immunity* and protect against infection with these or related organisms (i.e. produce *protective immunity*). See *anti idiotype vaccine, attenuated vaccine, heterologous carrier vaccines, inactivated vaccine, live vaccine, recombinant vaccine, smallpox vaccination, vaccination* and *adjuvant*.

vaccinia Synonym for the virus (*Poxvirus officinale*) formerly used in *vaccination* procedures to produce *immunity* to smallpox (variola) in man. Differs from the *cowpox* virus (*Poxvirus bovis*) and the smallpox virus (*Poxvirus variolae*) in minor *antigens* only, but was probably derived originally from cowpox virus.

valency (1) The valency of an *antibody* equals the number of *epitopes* to which one molecule of that antibody can bind. *IgG, IgD* and *IgE* have two *antigen-binding sites* and thus are divalent. *IgM* has 10 antigen-binding sites and *IgA* can exist as a monomer, dimer, trimer or tetramer having valencies of two, four, six and eight. In practice, antibodies often bind fewer *antigen* molecules than predicted by their valency due to steric hindrance, especially IgM which is relatively inflexible due to the absence of a *hinge region*. (2) The valency of an antigen may likewise be expressed as the number of epitopes it possesses. Most large antigen molecules are multivalent and therefore able to form large complexes with antibody at equivalence (see *optimal proportions*) due to the formation of a three dimensional lattice, see *lattice hypothesis*.

variable region (V-region) A sequence of approximately 115 amino acids at the N-terminus of the *light chain* (V$_L$) and the *heavy chain* (V$_H$) of *immunoglobulin* molecules and the α, β, γ and δ chains of the *TCR* (T cell receptor). The amino acid sequences in these regions are responsible for the great diversity of the *antigen-binding site* and T cell receptor *repertoires*, each clone of *B cells* or *T cells* producing molecules with different variable regions. This variation determines the conformation of the antigen-binding site and hence *antibody* specificity. The enormous variability of antibody molecules and TCRs is the result of random recombination events between the V exon, *D exon* and *J exon* occurring during the differentiation of a *stem cell* to a B or T lymphocyte. In B cells, further variability occurs during an immune response due to *somatic hypermutation* in the variable region. Many other members of the *Ig superfamily* contain domains homologous to the variable regions of immunoglobulin. See also *V-gene* and Figure I2.

variable region group The *variable regions* of *heavy chains* and *light chains* contain three *hypervariable regions* separated by *framework regions*. The framework regions show similarities in amino acid and base (DNA) sequence with other variable regions. These related sequences are placed within a group. Some groups are further divided into subgroups, see *variable region subgroup*.

variable region subgroup (1) Term used synonymously with *variable region group* q.v. to describe *variable regions* of human *immunoglobulins*. (2) Sufficient mouse V_κ variable region sequences have been determined to divide some of the variable region groups into subgroups, the members of which are more closely related in amino acid or base (DNA) sequence than other members of the same group.

variola (smallpox; variola major) An infectious disease caused by *Poxvirus variolae* and characterized by disfiguring vesicular and later pustular skin eruptions, viraemia and profound toxaemia. Now eliminated worldwide following WHO campaign.

vascular permeability factors Substances which increase the permeability of the walls of small vessels and thus enhance the passage of protein, cells, etc. from blood into the extra-vascular fluid. Include molecules such as *histamine, serotonin, kinins* and *leukotrienes*.

vasoactive amines Substances containing amino groups, such as *histamine* and *serotonin*, which cause peripheral vasodilation and increase the permeability of small vessels.

VCAM-1 (vascular cell adhesion molecule-1; CD106) A *Type I transmembrane protein* of the *Ig superfamily*, weakly expressed on normal vascular endothelium, but strongly expressed after exposure to *cytokines* such as IL-1, TNF-α and IL-4. VCAM-1 is a *ligand* for VLA-4 (*CD29/CD49*d) on *lymphocytes* and *monocytes*. VCAM-1 is also found on *dendritic cells*, including *interdigitating cells*, and thus probably contributes to lymphocyte–dendritic cell clustering in the induction of *immune responses*.

veiled cell A cell characterized by large veil-like processes; found in afferent *lymph* especially after *priming* with *antigen*. Veiled cells possess *accessory cell* function, and represent an intermediate stage between peripheral *dendritic cells* (e.g. *Langerhans cells*) and the dendritic cells of *lymphoid tissues* (e.g. *interdigitating cells*).

V_H **region** The *variable region* of the *heavy chain* of *immunoglobulin*.

virgin lymphocyte A *lymphocyte* that has not met *antigen*. An *unprimed* lymphocyte.

virus neutralization tests Tests used to measure *antibody* response to a virus or, vice versa, to identify the virus. Depends on the fact that specific antibody neutralizes the infectivity of viruses. They may be carried out *in vivo* in susceptible animals or chick embryos or, more usually, in tissue cultures. See *neutralization test*.

V_κ The *variable region* of the κ (kappa) *chain* of *immunoglobulin*.

V_L **region** The *variable region* of the *light chain* of *immunoglobulin*.

VLA-4 See *CD49*.

V_λ The *variable region* of the λ (lambda) *chain* of *immunoglobulin*.

W

Waldenström's macroglobulinaemia Disease occurring mainly in elderly males, characterized by proliferation of cells that make *monoclonal* IgM *paraprotein*. Serum *IgM* levels are high and there is *lymph node* enlargement, splenomegaly, a haemorrhagic tendency and hyperviscosity of blood. *Bone marrow* and *lymphoid tissues* are infiltrated with pleomorphic *lymphocytes* and *plasma cells*. Course of disease more benign than that of *myelomatosis*.

Wassermann reaction *Complement fixation test* used in the diagnosis of syphilis.

wasting disease Fatal disease developed by neonatally *thymectomized* animals and characterized by loss of weight, hunched appearance, ruffled fur and diarrhoea. *Germ free* neonatally thymectomized mice do not develop wasting disease, which has been taken as evidence that the impairment of *cell-mediated immunity* in thymectomized *conventional animals* leads to some form of fatal infection. However, neonatally thymectomized mice develop widespread multi-organ *autoimmunity* which may be the cause of the disease.

water-in-oil emulsion adjuvant An *adjuvant* in which the antigen, dissolved or suspended in water, is enclosed as tiny droplets within a continuous phase of mineral oil. The antigen solution constitutes the disperse phase. The phases are stabilized, so that they do not readily separate out, by the presence of an emulsifier such as Arlacel A® in the oil. See *incomplete Freund's adjuvant* and *complete Freund's adjuvant*.

weal and flare response Local response of skin to injury. Following minor, non-penetrating injury of any type or degree, erythema limited to the injured site appears immediately. This is followed in a minute or two by formation of a weal or oedema in the line of injury and a flare or erythema spreading out round the site. This was described by Thomas Lewis in 1927 as the 'triple response' and is due to release of *histamine*. Skin lesions of *immediate hypersensitivity* (*type I hypersensitivity reaction*) follow exactly the pattern described by Lewis and are due to the *IgE*-mediated release of histamine from *mast cells*.

Wegener's granulomatosis A severe necrotizing vasculitis involving especially the respiratory tract, kidney, joints and muscles. Tests for *anti neutrophil cytoplasmic antibody* are usually positive.

western blotting See *immunoblotting* which is the preferred term. The term 'western blotting' was coined to describe immunoblotting by analogy with *Southern blotting* and *northern blotting* used for the detection of DNA and RNA molecules.

wheat germ agglutinin A *lectin* q.v.

white cells The nucleated cells of the blood (i.e. *granulocytes, lymphocytes* and *monocytes*) so-called because they form a white layer over the erythrocytes when sedimented.

white pulp See *spleen*.

Wiskott–Aldrich syndrome X-linked *immunodeficiency* with low blood *platelet* count, bleeding, *eczema*, recurrent infections and a high incidence of *lymphomas* and epithelial tumours. There is defective *cell-mediated immunity* and absent *delayed-type hypersensitivity* reactions, and a defective *antibody* response to polysaccharide *antigens* with high serum *IgA* and *IgE* and low *IgM* levels. There is frequently deficient expression of *CD43* on *leucocytes*.

WR See *Wassermann reaction*

X

X-linked agammaglobulinaemia (Bruton-type hypogammaglobulinaemia) *Antibody deficiency syndrome* in boys which becomes manifest once maternally derived *antibodies* (see *maternal immunity*) have disappeared from the child's tissues. There are low numbers of circulating *B cells* and very low levels of all *immunoglobulins*. *Pre-B lymphocytes* are present in normal numbers in the *bone marrow*. Characterized by repeated, severe bacterial infections. There is a single defect in a gene on the X chromosome identified as *btk* (Bruton Tyrosine Kinase). This codes for a *protein tyrosine kinase* presumptively required for B cell maturation beyond the pre-B lymphocyte stage.

X-linked hyper-IgM syndrome X-linked recessive disease characterized by symptoms of *antibody* deficiency, e.g. pyogenic infections. *IgM*-producing *B cells* are present but *germinal centres* are not formed in response to foreign *antigens*. Patients lack the gene for *CD40L*, thus their *T cells* are unable to help B cells. The B cells fail to show *isotype switching* from IgM to *IgG* or *IgA in vivo* so that serum levels of IgM are high and of IgG and IgA are low.

X-linked lymphoproliferative syndrome (Duncan's syndrome) An X-linked lymphoproliferative condition in man, with uncontrolled proliferation of *B lymphocytes* producing tumours and rupture of the *spleen*. Caused by an *immune response* defect transmitted by the X chromosome so that the individual cannot resist Epstein–Barr virus infection (see *infectious mononucleosis*) in the normal way.

X-linked SCID (XSCID) see *SCID*.

xenogeneic (xenogenic; heterogeneic) Preferred term for grafted tissue that has been derived from a species different from the recipient. See also *transplantation terminology*.

xenograft (heterograft) Preferred term for a graft from a donor of dissimilar species.

xenotype Structural or antigenic difference between molecules, e.g. *immunoglobulins*, cell membrane *antigens*, etc., derived from different species.

xid **gene** A gene on the X chromosome in mice which codes for Btk, a *protein tyrosine kinase*. A mutation in this gene is present in CBA/N mice and causes an *immunodeficiency* similar to human *X-linked agammaglobulinaemia*.

Z

ZAP-70 (zeta chain associated protein) A *T cell, protein tyrosine kinase* that associates with the ζ *chain* following *TCR* stimulation. Mutations in the ZAP-70 gene are associated with some cases of *SCID*.

ζ (zeta) **chain** A 16 KD molecule that associates with the *CD3* molecule, and that plays a role in T cell receptor (*TCR*)-mediated signalling. Forms dimers either with another ζ chain or with an η (eta) chain. ζ chains are also associated with *Fc receptors* (CD16) and have homology with the γ chain of FcϵRI (see *Fcϵ receptors*).

zooprophylaxis The induction in man of *immunity* to a parasite by exposure to related parasites of lower animals, e.g. some degree of resistance to human schistosomiasis is produced by continual exposure to cercariae (the infective stage) of schistosomes of animals, such cercariae only producing abortive infections. Classic example was prevention of smallpox in man by vaccination with cowpox, see *Jennerian vaccination*.

zymosan Cell wall fraction of yeast (*Saccharomyces cerevisiae*) which activates the *alternative pathway* to *complement activation*, and thus binds *C3b*. Frequently used for study of opsonic (see *opsonin*) *phagocytosis*.

Appendix

Table 1 Standard Abbreviations

These abbreviations have been selected from the lists provided by several leading immunological journals and may, therefore, be considered standard at the time of writing.

Abbreviation	Item
Ab	antibody
Ag	antigen
AIDS	acquired immune deficiency syndrome
APC	antigen-presenting cell
BCG	bacille Calmette–Guérin
BM	bone marrow
BSA	bovine serum albumin
C	complement
C'	activated complement
C region	constant region (of Ig)
cDNA	complementary DNA
CDR	complementarity determining regions
CFA	complete Freund's adjuvant
CFU	colony-forming unit
CLL	chronic lymphocytic leukaemia
Con A	concanavalin A
CR	complement receptor
CSF	colony-stimulating factor
CTL	cytotoxic T lymphocyte
D	diversity
D region	diversity region of Ig or TCR
DNP	(2,4-)dinitrophenyl
DTH	delayed-type hypersensitivity
E	erythrocyte (e.g. E-rosette)
EAE	experimental allergic encephalomyelitis
EBV	Epstein–Barr virus
ELISA	enzyme-linked immunosorbent assay
Fab	Fab fragment
$F(ab')_2$	$F(ab')_2$ fragment
FACS	fluorescence activated cell sorter
FITC	fluorescein isothiocyanate
GM-CSF	granulocyte/macrophage colony-stimulating factor
GVH	graft-versus-host reaction
GVHD	graft-versus-host disease
H chain	heavy chain
HAT	hypoxanthine, aminopterin, thymidine
HIV	human immunodeficiency virus
HLA	human histocompatibility leucocyte antigen
HSA	human serum albumin
ID50	50% infective/inhibiting dose

IEF	isoelectric focusing
IFA	incomplete Freund's adjuvant
IFN	interferon (e.g. IFN-α)
Ig	immunoglobulin
IL	interleukin (e.g. IL-1)
Ir	immune response (e.g. Ir gene)
IU	International Unit
J	joining (e.g. J chain, J exon)
KLH	keyhole limpet haemocyanin
L chain	light chain
LAK	lymphokine-activated killer
LFA	lymphocyte function associated (e.g. LFA-1)
LGL	large granular lymphocyte
LN	lymph node
LPS	lipopolysaccharide
mAb	monoclonal antibody
MHC	major histocompatibility complex
MLC	mixed lymphocyte/leucocyte culture
MLR	mixed leucocyte reaction
Mls	minor lymphocyte stimulating (antigen)
MΦ	macrophage
NK cell	natural killer cell
NZB	New Zealand black mice
NZW	New Zealand white mice
OVA	ovalbumin
PAGE	polyacrylamide gel electrophoresis
PBL	peripheral blood lymphocyte
PBMC	peripheral blood mononuclear cell
PCA	passive cutaneous anaphylaxis
PCR	polymerase chain reaction
PE	phycoerythrin
PFC	plaque forming cell
PFU	plaque forming unit
PG	prostaglandins
PHA	phytohaemagglutinins
PKC	protein kinase C
PMN	polymorphonuclear leucocyte
PPD	purified protein derivative (of tuberculin)
PWM	pokeweed mitogen
r	recombinant (e.g. rIFN-γ)
R	receptor (e.g. IL-1R)
RBC	red blood cell (erythrocyte)
RF	rheumatoid factor
RFLP	restriction fragment length polymorphism (analysis)
RIA	radioimmunoassay
SCID	severe combined immunodeficiency (syndrome)
sIg	surface immunoglobulin
SLE	systemic lupus erythematosus
SRBC	sheep red blood cells
TCR	T cell receptor
TGF	transforming growth factor

Th   T helper cell
TNF   tumour necrosis factor
TRITC   tetramethylrhodamine isothiocyanate
Ts   T suppressor cell (suppressor T lymphocyte)
V region   variable region

Table 2   Single Letter Symbols for the Amino Acids

A	Alanine	G	Glycine	M	Methionine	S	Serine
C	Cysteine	H	Histidine	N	Asparagine	T	Threonine
D	Aspartic acid	I	Isoleucine	P	Proline	V	Valine
E	Glutamic acid	K	Lysine	Q	Glutamine	W	Tryptophan
F	Phenylalanine	L	Leucine	R	Arginine	Y	Tyrosine

Table 3   Greek Alphabet

This is shown in the Greek alphabetical order. Note that it is unusual for the upper case forms to be used in the biological sciences ($M\Phi$ is an exception) though these are shown for completeness.

Upper case	Lower case	English name under which the letters are alphabetized in this book
A	α	alpha
B	β	beta
Γ	γ	gamma
Δ	δ	delta
E	ε	epsilon
Z	ζ	zeta
H	η	eta
Θ	θ	theta
I	ι	iota
K	κ	kappa
Λ	λ	lambda
M	μ	mu
N	ν	nu
Ξ	ξ	xi
O	o	omicron
Π	π	pi
P	ρ	rho
Σ	σ	sigma
T	τ	tau
Y	υ	upsilon
Φ	φ	phi
X	χ	chi
Ψ	ψ	psi
Ω	ω	omega

The editors will be grateful to the readers for bringing to their attention any errors that they may find in the text and for suggestions and amendments. These should be sent to:

Professor P.C. Wilkinson
Department of Immunology
Western Infirmary
Glasgow, Scotland, G11 6NT
Fax 0141 337 3217